W9-AVJ-163

BUILT FOR SHOW

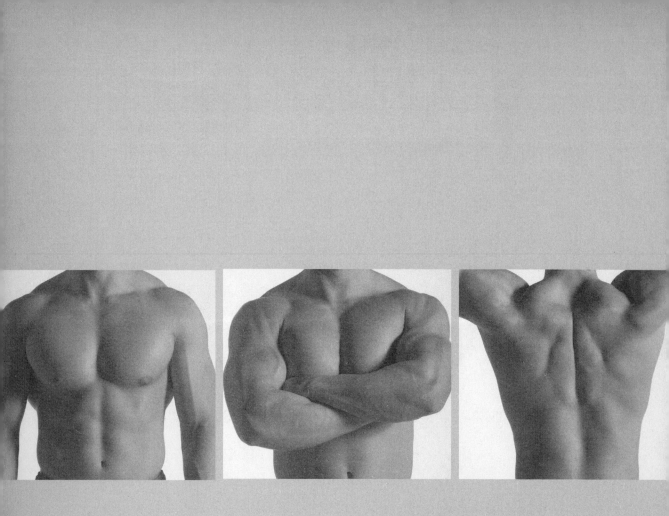

BUILT FOR SHOW

Four Body-Changing Workouts for Building Muscle, Losing Fat,
and Looking Good Enough to Hook Up

NATE GREEN

AVERY

a member of Penguin Group (USA) Inc.

New York

Published by the Penguin Group

Penguin Group (USA) Inc., 375 Hudson Street, New York, New York 10014, USA • Penguin Group (Canada), 90 Eglinton Avenue East, Suite 700, Toronto, Ontario M4P 2Y3, Canada (a division of Pearson Canada Inc.) • Penguin Books Ltd, 80 Strand, London WC2R 0RL, England • Penguin Ireland, 25 St Stephen's Green, Dublin 2, Ireland (a division of Penguin Books Ltd) • Penguin Group (Australia), 250 Camberwell Road, Camberwell, Victoria 3124, Australia (a division of Pearson Australia Group Pty Ltd) • Penguin Books India Pvt Ltd, 11 Community Centre, Panchsheel Park, New Delhi–110 017, India • Penguin Group (NZ), 67 Apollo Drive, Rosedale, North Shore 0632, New Zealand (a division of Pearson New Zealand Ltd) • Penguin Books (South Africa) (Pty) Ltd, 24 Sturdee Avenue, Rosebank, Johannesburg 2196, South Africa

Penguin Books Ltd, Registered Offices: 80 Strand, London WC2R 0RL, England

Most Avery books are available at special quantity discounts for bulk purchase for sales promotions, premiums, fund-raising, and educational needs. Special books or book excerpts also can be created to fit specific needs. For details, write Penguin Group (USA) Inc. Special Markets, 375 Hudson Street, New York, NY 10014.

Library of Congress Cataloging-in-Publication Data

Green, Nate.
Built for show : four body-changing workouts for building muscle, losing fat, and looking good enough to hook up / Nate Green.
p.   cm.
Includes bibliographical references and index.
ISBN 978-1-58333-319-8
1. Bodybuilding.   2. Physical fitness for men.   I. Title.
GV546.5.G74   2008   2008034870
613.7'13—dc22

Printed in the United States of America
1   3   5   7   9   10   8   6   4   2

BOOK DESIGN BY AMANDA DEWEY

ACKNOWLEDGMENTS

First, I must thank Lou Schuler for his guidance, honesty, and expertise. This book was just a simple idea before Lou took hold and made it a reality. Randomly e-mailing you five years ago was one of the best decisions I've ever made. I bow down to your writing skills and am thankful I've got you on my side.

Jason Lengstorf, you're an amazing friend who's always kept me in check. Together, I think we've solved most of the world's problems (while creating some of our own, of course). If I were gay, I'd possibly consider you my Tuesday boyfriend. Possibly.

Thanks to our collaborators on *Built For Show* for making the book better than I'd dared hope it would be: our editor, Megan Newman, and everyone at Avery; our agent, David Black; and our photographer, Michael Tedesco. Extra-special thanks go out to Mike Cerimele and the staff at Velocity Sports in Allentown, where we shot the photos, and to Jeff Hewlings and the trainers at the

Human Performance Center next door. We couldn't have asked for more cheerful or gracious cooperation than we got from Mike, Jeff, and their teams.

As a fitness guy in his early twenties, I've been helped by the guidance, generosity, and friendship of my fellow fitness professionals. In no particular order, I want to thank Alwyn Cosgrove, TC Luoma, Tim Patterson, Robert Dos Remedios, Eric Cressey, Mike Robertson, Craig Ballantyne, Sean Hyson, Adam Campbell, Bill Hartman, John Berardi, Chad Waterbury, Phill Fetlam, Mike Boyle, Charles Staley, Mike Roussell, Dan John, Josh Staph, Ryan Lee, Jim Labadie, Pat Rigsby, Craig Weller, Nick Berry, Joel Marion, Vince DelMonte, George Grigoryan, and everyone at *Men's Fitness, T-Nation, Men's Health, Maximum Fitness,* and *Stack.*

Thanks to Joel Bernstein for lending a hand personally and professionally. I'll have the Stella Artois on ice next time you visit. Thanks to Tim Ferriss, Ryan Holliday, Cindy Dyson, and all the other authors, Internet marketers, and general badasses I randomly e-mail for advice. And a big dose of gratitude goes out to my good friends, dedicated lifting partners and mentors in their own right: Kyle Hibler, Nate Steele, Dan Fern, Casey Becker, Sam Glauber, and Rob Farrington.

To all of my clients past, present, and future: thanks for trusting me with your bodies. And thanks to a very special group of clients who actually help me as much as I help them: Clay Bradley, Cary Collier, Diane Smith, Larry Cates, Kevin Smyley, Nancy LaRocque, and Dan Slezak.

This section wouldn't be complete without my thanking the most important people in my life: my parents; my brothers, Brian, Jordan, and Austin; and my grandpa. I love you all.

For my parents, Jeff and Janie Green, for teaching me it's not where you come from that's important. It's where you're going. Let's aim for the sky.

CONTENTS

Foreword by Lou Schuler   *xi*

PART 1. Cutting Through the B.S.

ONE. What a Guy *Really* Wants, and Why   *3*

TWO. You've Been Misinformed and Downright Lied To   *9*

THREE. The Bad, the Ugly, and the Uglier   *23*

PART 2. Building the Head-Turning Body

FOUR. The Goods, and How to Get Them   *41*

FIVE. Before You Start the Workouts . . .   *47*

SIX. Unlocking the Goods   *66*

SEVEN. The *Built for Show* Programs   *72*

EIGHT. The *Built for Show* Exercises   *99*

PART 3. Feeding, Clothing, and Showing Off the Body You've Built

NINE, These Foods Can Make or Break Your Physique   *183*

TEN, How to Flaunt What You Have and Hide What You Don't   *203*

ELEVEN. Presenting…You!   *214*

TWELVE. The End of the Beginning   *230*

Resources and Recommended Reading: The Other *Goods*   *233*

Index   *237*

FOREWORD

I have a confession to make: If you're reading this, I'm jealous of you. You may not know how lucky you are, but I do. You get a book that's targeted to your age group, specifically focused on the results you want most.

Me? When I started lifting in 1970, I was the skinniest thirteen-year-old I knew. I wanted the same results back then that you want now, adjusted for inflation. (In other words, I would've settled for any outcome that made me non-skinny; the idea of actually ending up "built for show" was beyond my wildest dreams.) I had never seen a bodybuilding magazine, much less a book explaining the nuances of strength training.

TV back then was five channels (three networks, PBS, and an independent station that ran *I Love Lucy* reruns), and if you think the Internet existed in 1970, I can only guess that the education system has left at least one child behind. The closest we got to physique-building instruction was the Charles Atlas ad in the back of our comic books. Of course, that was just a come-on to get us to send Atlas money; the pubescent male brain isn't noted for its consistent engagement with reality, but even at that modestly mindful age I suspected that "dynamic tension" would leave me poorer but no stronger.

I did get a few things right, almost by accident. I had no bench or power rack, so by necessity every exercise I did started with the weights on the floor. I did lots of push-ups and pull-ups, and my only regret is that I stopped doing them as a young adult when I finally got to work out in health clubs instead of my basement or garage.

Yes, I said it: Working out in commercial gyms, if anything, made my workouts worse instead of better. I suddenly had access to more equipment than I knew what to do with, and I mean that literally. I gravitated toward machines because they looked more interesting than free weights. I stopped doing pull-ups because lat pulldowns were more fun. I never did a squat or a deadlift—the exercises I now know are best for building a bigger, stronger, more athletic-looking body—because I had access to leg-extension, leg-curl, and leg-press machines. I may have even done a set or two on those leg-spreader and knee-slammer machines. I'd guess I performed five times as much upper-body work as I did for my lower body. Maybe ten times as much.

If I learned a new exercise for a set of muscles I hadn't yet targeted, I had to incorporate it into my workouts. It wasn't enough that I had exercises for my front, back, and middle deltoids. Those muscles actually exist, even if they don't need to be targeted with their own specialized exercises. I also had exercises for muscles that *don't* exist, like my upper and lower biceps and inner and outer pectorals.

As my young friend Nate Green might say, this is how skinny guys stay skinny.

My story has a happy ending: Because I started working at a fitness magazine in my mid-thirties, I learned enough about muscles to make mine grow. I could finally look in the mirror and see a guy who wasn't skinny, something I'd wanted since I was thirteen. The fact that I was middle-aged, bald, married, and raising girls instead of chasing them didn't really bother me. Muscles are cool at any age.

You, on the other hand, don't have to wait. With *Built for Show,* you have a book that's not only created for you, but also written by someone very much like you—and, for that matter, very much like me all those years ago. Nate may have figured things out at a much younger age than I did, but he's still someone who started with a desire to make a physical transformation. From his own experience and that of his clients, he knows how difficult it is to make dramatic and lasting changes in the way your body looks and performs. Under Nate's tutelage, you'll do the right exercises, employ the most effective training techniques, and make progress as fast as it can be made.

Did I mention that I'm jealous of you?

—*Lou Schuler*

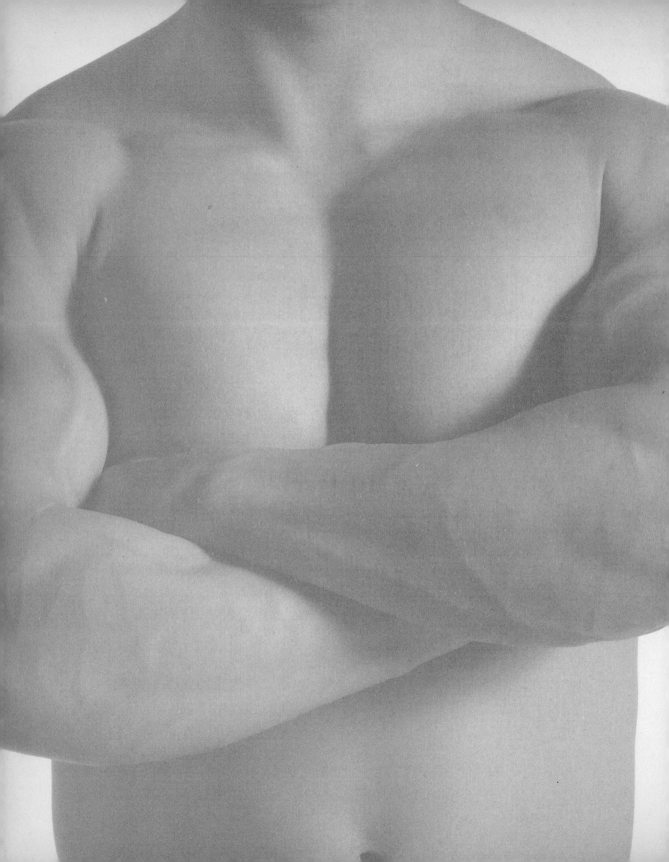

PART 1

Cutting Through the B.S.

CHAPTER ONE

What a Guy *Really* Wants, and Why

I'm going to ask you a question and I want you to give it to me straight. I've heard all sorts of answers from all sorts of guys, so my B.S. detector is finely tuned and has had quite a bit of practice. So I need you to level with me when you answer this question:

Why do you want to work out?

Why does *any* guy want to work out? Why train with weights at all?

If you said "to lower my cholesterol levels," "to touch the rim," or "to prevent osteoporosis later in life," I'm not buying it. There's nothing wrong with those benefits, and I'm sure you'll achieve them from the workouts I've designed. But come on. You don't lift because you're worried about your health or your performance in pickup basketball games.

You work out so you can increase your chances of hooking up. That means having the kind of physique that looks good in clothes and looks even better naked.

I'll accept variations on that answer. Like, "I go to the gym because my wife tells me to." Or, "If I don't stay in shape, my girlfriend will find someone who does." I know a few guys who won't even go to the grocery store if they don't look their best.

I get it. Some guys are born motivated, some achieve motivation, and some have motivation thrust upon them. But at the root of our motivation is an understanding that, when all else is equal, the guy with the better physique gets the girl. The combination of well-developed muscle mass and minimal body fat (what anthropologists mean when they report that the indigenous males of a particular region are "jacked") is a sign of reproductive fitness. It shows that you have more testosterone than the next guy, even if you don't. The more primed women are for sex, the more they notice. (True fact: Published scientific research shows that women are more attracted to the manliest men when they are ovulating than they are at other times in their menstrual cycle.) If you're Tarzan, she's game.

So let's start this relationship with some mutual candor. I wrote this book because nobody else did. There was a time, not long ago, when I wanted to know more about building my body in hopes of accumulating more frequent-fornication points. I wanted exactly what you want: muscles that women notice. I couldn't find that book, because it wasn't yet written. Instead, I learned how to achieve the goal, and in the process became a very busy personal trainer. Then I set out to write the book I always wanted to read.

That's enough about me. Let's talk about you.

Whether you're thick or thin, you want the wide shoulders and chiseled torso that women don't just notice, they occasionally grab. You don't wish bodily harm on anybody, but you'd be flattered to know that the woman who just passed you on the freeway risked soft-tissue damage when her head whipped around to get a better look.

At a bare minimum, you want the most attractive women in your apartment complex to see you as the go-to guy the next time they need some furniture moved.

Now that we've cleared the air about why you want the body you want, let's talk about something a bit more complex: Why don't you have that kind of body already? I'm going to assume you're familiar with the concept of working out. If I were a betting man, I'd wager that most of you reading this work out regularly. But if you're like most of the guys I see in gyms these days, you're doing workouts that can't possibly help you reach your goals.

Worse, I see some of the finest young men of my generation exercising in a way that will take them further away from their goals. Some of the more sharp-tongued members of my profession refer to commercial gyms as "fatness centers." Health clubs encourage you to come in and mope your way through useless circuits on machines that only exist as marketing tools to make strength training look "easy" to the newbies. They discourage you from working hard by making it relatively inconvenient to do the exercises that build the most muscle mass. One gym chain on the East Coast even has a rule against grunting. I'm as opposed to gratuitous noise as anybody, but how do you push yourself to get stronger if you have to worry about getting kicked out of the damned gym just because an exertion-related sound involuntarily escaped from your throat?

There are lots of ways to work out that don't involve the risk of breathing hard. That's why the health-club chains want you to do high-repetition, low-weight circuits on their shiny exercise machines. You won't build the body you want with those workouts, but the owners of the health clubs don't care. They're happy to see you waste your time, as long as your account is paid in full.

Frankly, though, I couldn't care less about people who want results without hard work. I'm more concerned with the guys who work hard but don't ever get the results they've earned. I see a lot of these lifters falling into three distinct categories:

BODY BY *FLEX*

These are the guys who "blast their biceps" with thirty-two different exercises, following the workouts of the pro bodybuilders they read about in the magazines. They never ask if their biceps need to be blasted at all, much less with thirty-two exercises. Result? Their muscles get more blood-engorged than a tick with a rather serious glandular problem, but once the blood drains back out of their biceps the result is . . . deflating.

GHOST OF WORKOUTS PAST

Remember the workout program you did in high school, back when you put on twenty pounds of solid muscle your senior year, when you made third-team all-conference? Your muscles sure as hell remember. That's why you haven't gotten any stronger since high school. It was probably a great workout (although I've seen some pretty crappy programs designed by high school coaches). Still, no matter how well designed the program was, a body will make only so many adaptations to any one system of training. Without variety, there's no challenge. Without challenge, there's no progress.

IF IT'S NEW, IT MUST BE BETTER

It's great to be open-minded about new ideas in training. But it can go too far. The smartest, most successful trainers I know make endless fun of the people balancing on Bosu balls while attempting to lift weights that are too light to put muscle on the glandular tick I mentioned a moment ago. (A Bosu ball is half of a rubber ball on top of a plastic platform. Consider yourself lucky if you've never encountered one.) Unless you're training to be an acrobat, it's far better to work out with one or both feet on the floor, since that's the way you use your muscles in real life.

Most guys I see end up doing workouts that are hybrid versions of all the pitfalls I just described. It's not that they don't have enough information. Between books, magazines, and the Internet, there's more information than ever. And if it was as good as it claims to be, we'd all be ripped to shreds and warming up on the bench press with five hundred pounds.

The information itself is often the problem, especially when it comes from the wrong sources: muscle magazines, misinformed personal trainers, Hollywood "trainers to the stars" . . . sometimes the stars themselves pretend to be fitness experts. The truth is that most "fitness experts" have no idea how to get actual results for actual humans.

That's why a typical guy's workout looks something like this:

STEP ONE: Walk into gym.

STEP TWO: Bench-press, incline bench-press, dumbbell bench-press, dumbbell incline bench-press, hop on a treadmill.

STEP THREE: Try to impress the girl on the machine next to you by flexing your pecs while you run.

STEP FOUR: Go home alone and cry.

STEP FIVE: Return to the gym the next day, only instead of twenty-four sets of chest exercises, you do twenty each for your biceps and triceps. And instead of flexing your pecs while you run on the treadmill, you flex your arms, making you look like you're auditioning for a remake of *Robocop*.

That's why I wrote *Built for Show*. If you have the motivation and desire, you deserve a program that shows you how to reach your goals, step-by-step. You deserve a system that makes efficient use of your time and energy.

I hope you get a little more knowledgeable about training when you read *Built for Show*. (I know I got a lot smarter writing it. You never know what you don't know until you try to verify the things you *think* you know.) And I'm sure you'll get a lot of benefits that don't matter much to you now. You'll build stronger bones, lowering your risk of osteoporosis. You'll ramp up your metabolism, making it easier to keep body fat from returning, or from accumulating in the first place. If you have some nagging little injuries, you'll probably find they become a lot less bothersome.

All of those are perfectly nice side effects, like going on *The Price Is Right* and winning a coffeemaker as a consolation prize when you were hoping for the convertible Mustang. My guess is that you wouldn't be very consoled. But if you won the grand prize, you wouldn't complain about finding the coffeemaker in the backseat.

Are you ready to go after that grand prize?

ABOUT THE PROGRAMS

I'll get into this in much greater detail in Chapter 7, but right now you're probably curious about what you'll be doing to get built for show. My yearlong workout system is divided into four seasonal programs:

Fall: I hope most readers will start here, especially those who haven't yet spent a lot of time in the weight room. These workouts introduce you to the most important exercises, like squats and deadlifts, and focus on building a base of strength and muscle mass while providing enough of a training stimulus to work off a little fat in the process.

Winter: Here you'll focus on building pure strength, which also packs muscle on the places where women will notice it.

Spring: The goal here is to continue building your strength and muscle size while also making your workouts more challenging. So you'll improve your overall conditioning and athleticism while burning off some fat and getting your body ready for display.

Summer: Now you'll seriously attack whatever remaining fat you have with more technically complex exercises and tougher workouts. You'll also get to do some curls and extensions to put the finishing touches on your physique.

The system is modular, so you can start with any program that suits your needs and is compatible with your current abilities. I encourage most of you to start at the beginning and continue for a year. It doesn't matter if you end up with your "summer" body in October or April; once you're built for show you'll reap the benefits any day of the year.

CHAPTER TWO

You've Been Misinformed and Downright Lied To

When I was six, I used to ask my parents probing questions.

"Why is the sky blue?" I asked. "Why does ice float?" "Why is that girl on TV so skinny? And why do they keep saying she's rich? If she had money, wouldn't she buy a sandwich?"

You know, important stuff any kid would want to know.

I also remember how they would shift uncomfortably in their chairs and roll their eyes at each other before smiling and giving me condescending answers:

"Because it'd look weird if it was red." "Because ice is cold and wants to get closer to the sun to get warm." "Because the richer a woman is, the less she's expected to eat. Now go outside and play with your firecrackers."

They had absolutely no idea how to answer me, but, being my parents, they felt obliged to tell me *something*. Too bad that something helped me flunk eighth-grade science and landed me on the U.S. Postal Service's watch list for trying to mail a half-dozen ham sandwiches to California. But that's another story.

People in the fitness industry, like my parents, make mistakes. They say things that aren't true, recommend things that aren't useful, and pretend to have expertise they don't actually have. Sometimes they have good intentions. Unlike my parents, though, they're getting paid to give advice and address your concerns. They don't refund your money if their recommendations don't work. They don't even let you stay up a half hour past bedtime because they feel guilty about misleading you. And worst of all, they keep making the same faulty recommendations long after they've been discredited.

My goal with this chapter is to look at some of the more pernicious training issues I see in my travels, explain why they persist, and, most important of all, explain why you deserve better.

THE PROBLEM: TOO MANY "BODY PARTS," NOT ENOUGH BODY

I call it the "body-part split epidemic"—BPSE for short. It's a technique that migrated downwind from professional bodybuilders like Arnold Schwarzenegger, who used to brag about doing dozens of sets for his biceps and triceps in a single workout. I don't know if Arnold actually did anything so extreme, or if he just said he did to trick his competitors into overtraining.

Either way, the advice filtered down from competitive bodybuilders to serious gym rats to senior citizens entering a gym for the first time. Just about everyone you see in any gym or weight room believes that it takes a lot of redundant movements to build muscles, and that each muscle you want to build has to be targeted with exercises specific to that particular "body part."

BPSE shows up in many forms.

Guys like us might have an "arm day" each week, in which they do nothing but exercises for their biceps and triceps. "Arm day" follows "chest day," "back day," and "shoulder day," but usually precedes "leg day." (This system of priorities leads to what I call "KFC syndrome," which I'll describe in a bit.)

Middle-aged guys with less time to train won't devote an entire workout to arm exercises. They'll just waste half of one each week doing curls and extensions.

Even old ladies with less than two weeks of training experience spend a quarter of their gym time on the triceps-pushdown station in a valiant (if futile) effort to "tone" the sagging flesh on their upper arms.

Sometimes guys with BPSE combine muscle groups in a way that makes you think some higher-level reasoning went into their workout philosophy. Let's say you ask one what his training schedule looks like for the week. (This question, by the way, is 100 percent effective in diagnosing BPSE.) "Well, I've got chest and triceps today," a typical gym rat might answer. "Then back and biceps tomorrow, legs and shoulders on Thursday, and forearms and abs on Friday."

It sounds like there's a sensible system in place. The triceps, after all, work together with the chest and shoulders when you do exercises like bench presses. The biceps work with the big upper-back muscles on lat pulldowns and rows. Even working "shoulders" with "legs" has a smidgen of logic, since the trapezius— the muscle that pulls the shoulder blades in several different directions—works with your gluteals and hamstrings on the deadlift. I can't think of a reason to do "forearms" and abs on the same day, but maybe that's just me. (For that matter, I can't really think of a reason to work forearms at all, in isolation, since they play important roles in every exercise worth doing.)

My point is, it makes sense when they describe it. It stops making sense if you ask why working a bunch of muscles in isolation is better than working them all at once.

A lot of the guys with BPSE are built well enough to make you think it's working for them. I'll freely acknowledge that some of them are bigger than me, and in better shape than a lot of the trainers and strength coaches who think this approach is misguided. Still, in my experience, most guys exhibiting symptoms of BPSE would be better off keeping it simple by working all their muscles each workout, emphasizing the exercises that use the most muscle mass in coordinated action, instead of trying to see how many exercises they can do for the smallest pieces of contractile tissue in isolation.

Well, How Did We Get Here?

Up until the 1950s, most bodybuilders did total-body workouts. Whether they were champions or wannabes working out with mail-order weight sets in their parents' garage, the most popular training method was to do three total-body workouts a week. It allowed a lifter to stimulate maximum muscle growth, and gave him just enough time to recover in between workouts.

Then came anabolic steroids.

Steroids encouraged bodybuilders to annihilate their muscles with more sets and reps than ever before, allowing them to grow to gargantuan proportions. The amazing thing about steroids is that the more you take, the better they work. Since their muscles could now do more work and recover faster from that work, bodybuilders had an incentive to invent more muscle-isolating exercises and exercise systems. As long as they took more muscle-building drugs, they could do more muscle-building exercises.

Unfortunately, nonsteroid users looked at these enormous men and thought it must be the training that produced those oversize chassis. Guys who were relative novices would see a pro bodybuilder's workout in *Muscle & Fitness* or *Flex* and think that's what they should do.

The first personal trainers were often former or aspiring bodybuilders, so they were on board with body-part splits. And, to make the circle complete, commercial gyms were designed to accommodate BPSE. You rarely see a free-weight area in a health club that's set up for heavy lifting, but you can always find rows of benches in front of the dumbbell rack, which is perfect for grinding out sets of curls and extensions.

Given all that, it's no surprise that most people in most gyms believe there's no better system, even though it works best for people taking steroids. The other 99 percent of the population are just setting themselves up for failure right from the start. They'd be better off training the way the old-timers used to do it.

Back to Basics

Imagine this: Your best friend calls to tell you he's just bought a 1966 Pontiac GTO, fire-engine red—a true classic. He asks you to come over to help him detail it. You walk over to his house, imagining that you're going to put a little more sparkle onto a machine that's already a work of art.

Then you walk into his garage and find a heap of oxidized metal propped up on cinder blocks. How the *hell* are you supposed to detail something that has more rust than paint?

Corny analogy aside, the average guy trying to build an attention-grabbing body needs to focus on the basics. Just as you can't detail a car that's three-quarters rust, you can't put the finishing touches on a body that's not yet built.

I believe the best, fastest, and most efficient way to build that body is with total-body training. I base this mostly on the results I've seen with my clients, my own success, and the training recommendations of my fellow fitness professionals. But I also believe that working your body as an integrated whole—doing exercises like squats, deadlifts, chin-ups, rows, and presses—makes intuitive sense. Your muscles evolved to work with one another in coordinated action, so why wouldn't you train them that way?

Here's a test to illustrate what I mean. Grab a pen and drop it on the ground. Now, try to pick it up using only one muscle. See what I mean? Let's try it again, but this time take stock of how many muscles really are working when you pick it up as you normally would. You bend, twist, and extend all kinds of muscles to reach down to the floor, and then you do the opposite of all those motions to return to whatever position you were in initially.

My point is that so many muscles work together to complete the simplest tasks that it's futile to try to isolate them. Imagine if that pen you just picked up had been a barbell. You couldn't possibly lift it off the floor with isolated muscle contractions—you'd activate muscles from your big toes to your pinky fingers to pick it up. The strongest muscles in your thighs and hips would have to work with the stabilizing muscles in your midsection to keep your spine where it's supposed to be. The bigger muscles in your shoulder area—delts, pecs, lats, and traps—have to provide a platform for the smaller muscles in your arms, and the muscles in your arms have to provide logistical support for the smaller muscles in your hands.

By the time you've performed the seemingly simple task of bending over, grabbing the bar, and then standing up again, you've activated hundreds of individual muscles, countless square feet of connective tissues, and trillions of nerve cells. Even if you plan to do an "isolation" exercise with that barbell once you lift it off the floor, such as a biceps curl, you can't possibly cut everything else out of the exercise and work nothing but your biceps. The muscles in your fingers, hands, and forearms are still holding on to the bar. The shoulder-area muscles are still working to provide your upper arms with a stable platform. The midsection muscles can't take a breather—your spine couldn't keep you upright without their effort. The lower-body muscles, from your glutes to your toes, have to do something to keep you vertical.

That said, here's a question that perplexed me when I was starting out as a trainer, and listened as the top guys in my field advised against doing exercises like biceps curls: how else can I build my biceps, or help my clients build theirs, if I don't do specialized biceps-building exercises? What could possibly take the place of direct biceps stimulation?

You can answer the question for yourself by grabbing onto the chin-up bar and pulling yourself up a few times. If you can't do that, try underhand-grip rows or pulldowns. Your biceps are working just as hard on those exercises, but they're also working synchronously with lots of other muscles, particularly those in your upper back. In fact, they're probably working *harder* on these pulling exercises, since the weights you're moving are heavier than the ones you'd use for curls.

You'll also notice that the movement is exactly the same, as far as your biceps are concerned. Your biceps are designed to bend your elbows, and that's exactly what you do on rows and chin-ups. How can the muscle fibers in your upper arms distinguish between exercises that are supposed to make them work in "isolation" versus exercises that include other muscle groups? If the movement is the same, and the workload is at least equal, why wouldn't the pulldowns and rows accomplish the same result?

So focusing on your big muscles, and cutting the isolation exercises from your workouts, saves you time. If you can get the same results with three hours a week in the gym, why would you want to spend more time there? Beyond the efficiency factor, total-body workouts help you reach your goals better than isolation exercises in three more ways:

- They burn more fat, since they take a lot of energy to perform, and keep your metabolism elevated for hours or even days after your workout.
- They cause your body to produce more of its muscle-building hormones.
- Because they use your muscles in coordinated actions, they contribute to a more athletic appearance. Even if you couldn't hit the ball out of the infield, you still wouldn't mind looking like the guy who can hit the long ball.

All this leads to another question: Do you *really* get the same results when you cut the curls and extensions out of your workouts? Isn't there an added benefit to doing those isolation exercises *in addition to* the deadlifts and squats and rows and presses?

If you were a competitive bodybuilder, I'd say yes, there's clearly some benefit to doing extra work for those muscles, even if you're drug-free. That's because competitive bodybuilders need to use every muscle-building trick in the book to stay competitive. A few extra centimeters of muscle here or there could be the difference between winning and losing.

But if you really are a competitive bodybuilder, you're reading the wrong book. I advise you to return it for a full refund. As much as I'd love to have your money, I can't take it in good conscience. I didn't write this book for you, and I would never pretend to be an expert in your sport.

For everyone else, remember the point I made earlier: unless you already have a head-turning physique, you don't need to worry so much about the details.

THE PROBLEM: YOU DON'T WORK WHAT YOU CAN'T SEE

Guys have a tendency to stick to what they're good at, and avoid everything else. That's why I kept playing T-ball through high school. And that's why most guys in most gyms spend most of their time doing their favorite exercises. Curiously, though, their favorite exercises are always the ones that work muscles they can see in a mirror. I have yet to meet a guy who tells me how much he likes doing chin-ups or bent-over barbell rows. But I've met plenty who boast about how much they can bench-press.

Of course, a good PR in the bench press is worth bragging about, and it's a perfectly fine standard to use when you're measuring yourself against other powerlifters.

If, however, you're not a powerlifter, then you have to ask yourself why the bench press is such a popular exercise, and why it's almost always the first exercise in the first workout of the week for lifters. The answer isn't difficult: it works the biggest muscles on the front of your body, the ones you notice first when you look in a mirror.

That's why so many guys are so good at it—and why even the guys who aren't good at it still do it first in their Monday workouts.

Meanwhile, the muscles that aren't easy to see in a mirror, the ones below your waist and behind your ribs, get left behind.

Well, How Did We Get Here?

Blame vanity. We all want to look in a mirror and feel good about what we see. It's why we shave, pay other people to cut our hair, and do biceps curls and abdominal crunches. If you want to think about how vanity affects the parts of our lives that we can't see in the bathroom mirror, ask yourself why guys like us go up to our eyeballs in debt to buy nicer cars than we can afford.

Because we're so often at the mercy of our most shallow needs, the fitness media have learned to exploit the situation. You could run out of fingers counting the references to abs and biceps on the covers of muscle magazines on any given newsstand in any given month, but you'll almost never see a reference to hamstrings on those covers.

I'm not exactly taking the high ground here. Vanity is fine with me. I can live with mine, and I sold you this book to help you act on yours. But I do want you to think about your vanity in a different way. I want you to consider *what other people see* when they look at you.

Sure, they see your pecs and delts and upper arms. If you have abs, and you happen to be shirtless, and you remember to stand just right, and it's not pitch-dark, they can see those as well. But they can also see your back, butt, and hamstrings. You may not know what you look like from the vantage point of someone standing directly behind you, but that doesn't mean you're invisible from that angle.

Believe me, if you have the dreaded KFC syndrome—pumped-up chest, chickenlike legs—women will notice. And my guess is that they won't like what they see.

You should also know that the women checking you out aren't wondering about the size of your bench press. Strength is good, of course, but only when it helps you reach your ultimate goal of a body that looks beautiful in the eye of your beholder. If your ego pushes you toward a bigger bench press at the expense of that ultimate goal . . . well, keep reading.

Back to Basics

My purpose here isn't to make you more self-conscious. I just want to help you look good to a potential partner, from whatever angle she happens to be looking at you.

That's why the workouts in *Built for Show* are balanced from top to bottom and front to back. You'll put the same effort into your lower-body muscles as you do the ones above the belt—no KFC syndrome allowed. You'll do equal amounts of pulling and pushing exercises, with equal intensity. As often as not, you'll do your least favorite exercises—the ones that work what I call the "reverse mirror muscles"—first in your workouts, to ensure that you do the most important work when you have the most strength and energy.

Another benefit to balanced workouts is that they help you overcome some of the hits you take in the cubicle farms where so many of us earn our beer money. We sit hunched over steering wheels on the way to work, we sit hunched over laptops when we're on the clock, we repeat the steering-wheel hunch on the way home, and then we spend a couple more hours each evening hunched over the laptop again.

It's not your imagination that your posture suffers from all this hunching. (This is what your parents were trying to prevent when they told you to sit up straight. And if you'd listened, it might've worked.) What happens is that the muscles on the front of your torso, your pecs mostly, get shorter and tighter. The muscles on the back of your torso get longer and looser. It also happens below the belt. Your hip flexors, those strips of muscle on the front of your pelvis, tighten up. The muscles behind them stretch out, which flattens the natural curve of your lower back, giving you the dreaded "buttless" look. That is, the top of your pelvis shifts backward, the bottom of it is pulled forward, and your butt cheeks end up shifting downward in shame.

People in my field who're older and smarter than me could tell you that the length-tension relationship of those muscles has been altered—some too short and tense, some stretched out and flaccid. Each muscle that loses its optimal length and level of tension pulls something else out of its ideal shape.

Now imagine that you, in an effort to improve your physique, overemphasize your pecs and abs in your workouts, when compared to the amount of work you give the muscles behind them. In pursuit of a brawnier bench press and more manageable midsection, you force those muscles to be shorter and tighter than they should be—compounding the problem created by all the other posture-wrecking things you do working and commuting. You're exacerbating the very problems you should be correcting in your workouts.

Not alarmed? Think of it this way: Suppose some hideous affliction made your penis shrink when you had an erection, but lengthen when you didn't have one. The phrase "Sucks to be you!" comes to mind, doesn't it?

So the solution takes care of multiple problems. You stand up straighter, more like an action hero than an ape. And you'll never have to worry about being called "buttless."

THE PROBLEM: YOU TRY TO SUPPLEMENT WHAT YOU DON'T YET HAVE

I like nutritional supplements. I use a bunch of them. I read about them constantly, and I have lots of experience with them. But because I own a dictionary, I also know that a "supplement" is "something added, especially to make up for a lack or deficiency." So you have vitamin supplements to help bridge the gap between what you generally eat and what your body needs. You have liquid protein supplements to make sure you get muscle-building nutrients at exactly the right time to do you the most good. And you have fish-oil supplements to make sure you get a beneficial fat that, unfortunately, has mostly disappeared from our diets.

Not one of these supplements will work as well as it's supposed to if the rest of your diet is crap.

Well, How Did We Get Here?

We've all seen the ads, featuring professional bodybuilders wearing their shiny, steroid-built muscles like knights showing off their new suits of armor. We've all been in GNC and seen the shelves of powders and pills. We all know the guys in gyms who swear one protein supplement is vastly superior to another.

And we've all gotten the message, one way or another, that nutritional supplements have almost magical powers to do for us what diet and training can't.

I agree with part of the message (not, obviously, the "magical" part). But I add this caveat: most of us have no idea how much we can do with diet and training—how much muscle we can build with a good diet and smart workouts, or how lean we can be without using anything with the words "fat burner" on the label.

Going even further, every smart person I've met in the strength and conditioning business will tell you, one way or another, that there's no real substitute for a good diet. Even guys who take steroids will get fat if they don't eat right.

Granted, they'll be fat with arms as big around as your thighs, but they won't be built for show. Not even close.

Back to Basics

I won't get into the details here—you'll find those in Chapter 9—but I will say this: if you want to be lean, you have to eat clean. With enough food, anyone can be big. You just have to lift a fork as relentlessly as you lift barbells and dumbbells. Food builds muscles but, if used indiscriminately, it also builds fat. It's a blunt instrument. No matter how many steaks you eat or how many supplements you take, the crap in your diet will prevent you from looking the way you want to look.

There's no single way to "eat clean." You can eat clean on a super-low-carb Atkins-type diet, on a low-fat vegetarian diet, or on anything in between. What you can't get away with is liquid calories in the form of Mountain Dew or the type of grease that clings to deep-fried chicken wings. The only thing wonderful about Wonder Bread is its ability to hit your bloodstream so fast you may as well have injected its carbohydrates directly into your veins.

And beer? It's against my personal code to tell you not to have something that I personally consume. But we both realize it's no accident that the word "belly" follows "beer" as often as it does. I won't tell you not to have an occasional cold one with your crime dogs, but I will suggest that the less beer you have, the more you'll enjoy it.

THE PROBLEM: YOU KNOW YOU'RE NOT A CHARACTER IN THE HARRY POTTER BOOKS, BUT YOU STILL BELIEVE IN MAGIC

When we walk into the weight room, determined to build a body that looks the way we want it to look, most of us are happy to leave reality outside in the cold, where it can't intrude on our dreams and desires for the next hour or so. Part of that escape is to imagine that we can shape specific parts of our bodies to match our society's fitness icons. You want abs like Brad Pitt. Biceps like Arnold. Maybe shoulders like LeBron.

Which, of course, is fine. It feels good to feel inspired . . . as long as you understand, once you're back out in the real world, what can and can't be done. Even the best workout and diet plan won't make you look like someone or something that your genes can't possibly conjure. You know you can't turn your eyes a different color or make yourself five inches taller or reverse a receding hairline. So you should realize that you can't turn the body your parents created into a mirror image of a body that emerged from the coupling of an entirely unrelated egg and an equally foreign sperm cell.

Well, How Did We Get Here?

I hate to keep picking on the fitness media, but it's unavoidable: who else gives us the idea that we can look like a famous athlete or bodybuilder or celebrity if we just do that person's workout?

Back to Basics

Every guy who works out wonders, at some point, why the program isn't doing what he expected.

"I did all the arm exercises the trainer said I need to do. Why don't my biceps have a peak like Arnold's?"

"I lost so much fat that my shoes fall off my feet unless I have on two pairs of socks. So how come I still can't see my abs?"

"I work out like a maniac for two weeks, just like the article in *Flex* said I should, but then I feel so run-down I can't even think about training for a week. Why can't I work out hard all the time?"

All these questions have the same answer: every aspect of training is influenced, to greater or lesser degrees, by our genes.

Most of us, for example, suspect that our relative ability or inability to work hard and recover fast is somehow related to the size of our testicles. If only we'd sack up, and act like real men, we could do more in the gym, and get there more often. You hear this from great athletes all the time: they'll thank God for their talent, but give themselves sole credit for the hard work they put in to exploit the talent. The truth is, they may be giving the Almighty too much credit for the former and not enough for the latter. Any of us can get into better shape, but some genetically gifted individuals will always be able to work harder than their peers, and recover faster from their workouts.

Similarly, any of us can make muscles bigger and make fat deposits smaller. But our genetic code determines the end result. Thus, even the best workout and diet ever devised can't take the final layer of fat off a belly that won't allow it. And it gets even worse than that: some guys who aren't particularly lean will still have defined abs, thanks to genetic programming that prevents fat from accumulating in the center of their abdominal region. Meanwhile, muscles that get bigger assume whatever shape your genetic code tells them to assume. Two of us can do the exact same workouts with the exact same effort, but our muscles will look vastly different at any given point in time.

Bodybuilding magazines wouldn't be complete without the articles on how to bring up your "lagging" body parts. But the best-conditioned and most knowledgeable bodybuilders you'll ever meet still have muscles that aren't the ideal size or shape. Some guys can build huge biceps and deltoids but get stuck with relatively puny calves. Others might have fantastically thick arms and legs, but relatively narrow shoulders. It's not because they aren't trying or don't know what they're doing. Their genes simply don't allow the "lagging" muscle groups to catch up to the ones that grow more easily.

That's yet another reason why I prescribe balanced workouts in *Built for Show.* By working everything important and neglecting nothing that matters, you'll get the best body your ancestors allow you to have.

CHAPTER THREE

The Bad, the Ugly, and the Uglier

We all start at the beginning. Where we end up depends a great deal on how we think of ourselves and the individual choices we make. Common sense, right?

But here's the part most people overlook: it's not the situation that's important. It's how you react to the situation. If you doubt yourself, make excuses, or succumb to procrastination and apathy, all you're doing is building a ceiling over yourself that will abruptly halt your progress before it even begins. And thumping your head against an immovable object is about as much fun as it sounds.

I used to be a skinny, shy little twerp who constantly sought approval from others to validate my life. But after defining the problem, trying to move past my limitations, blaming other people, cursing, making a lot of stupid mistakes, cursing even more (which, I confess, I mostly enjoy), and ultimately learning from my mistakes, I realized that I—and I alone—decided my individual outcome.

This was a sobering thought, and it brought about an epiphany: *Everything that happened to me was both my fault and* not *my fault.*

Lost yet? Let me put it another way.

Genetics matter, as I noted in Chapter 2, and they most definitely aren't your fault. But if you spend a lot of time thinking about the crap genes your parents handed you, and using them as an excuse for not reaching whatever goals you have, you've probably assigned them more power than they actually have. There isn't a scientist on earth who'd claim that 100 percent of your weight and shape are predetermined. A few weight-loss bloggers, maybe, but no actual scientists.

Training and diet matter, too, and that's what we're focusing on here. The *BFS* training program and nutritional guidelines are designed to alter what nature intended for you, as much as it can be altered. If you choose to follow the program, you're acknowledging both realities: you're changing what you can while recognizing that you can't completely reengineer your genome.

I absolutely can't tell you how much you can change. I've never worked with a client who couldn't put on muscle and take off fat. Every client has emerged from our training looking and feeling better—dramatically better, in many cases. But there's never a single pattern. Sometimes people achieve more than I expected, and I'm happy to take credit. But sometimes they achieve less, and if I'm willing to take credit for the overachievers I have to accept blame when a client falls below our mutual expectations.

What I can predict is that your success will be directly correlated with the effort you put in. And I'm not just talking about physical effort. You also have to change your attitude toward your own body and your preconceived ideas about its limitations. The following is by no means a complete list of attitudes that hold guys back, but it's a pretty good overview of the ones I see most often in friends and clients.

THINGS SKINNY GUYS BELIEVE THAT KEEP THEM SKINNY

"If I Eat More Calories, I'll Lose my Abs"

The skinny guy with well-defined abs often calls himself a "hard gainer." That is, he sees himself as a guy who can't create bigger muscles no matter how hard he tries. But this type of lifter often refuses to try the most logical solution to his problem: eating enough food to build the muscles he wants.

If you're truly a hard gainer—one of those guys whose metabolism resembles a hummingbird hooked on trailer-park meth—you need a dramatic increase in calories. Trust me, I've been there. As a 145-pound eighteen-year-old, my fork was my version of an American Express card: I couldn't leave home without it.

The good news is that the weight you gain will mostly be in the form of muscle. That's what happens when you have a fast metabolism; your body resists storing fat even more than it resists adding muscle.

But here's a concept few people in or out of the fitness business truly understand or apply: if you already have a fast metabolism, eating more food will actually make it *faster*. So the more food you eat, the less fat you accumulate. A lot of the excess calories will get burned off in this metabolic frenzy, but enough will get to your muscles to make a noticeable difference.

Thus, if you have abs before you start this muscle-growth program, you'll still have them when you finish.

"I Need to Do High Reps to Get More Definition"

This type of talk makes me want to at least partially blame the triathletes and marathon runners who use weight lifting as supplemental exercise, but don't understand the basics of exercise physiology. Performing hundreds of calf raises and triceps pushdowns while wearing latex shorts and skintight shirts will not make them or you "more defined." It gives your muscles a nice pump, but that's all.

What's wrong with that?

The science is pretty clear on this point: a pump doesn't make your muscles bigger, any more than standing on your head makes you smarter. It's just a bunch of blood in your muscles—good for your ego, but meaningless to your long-term muscular development. It comes, it temporarily stretches your shirt-sleeves, and then it goes.

The science also tells us this about muscle fibers: they can get bigger, they can get smaller, or they can stay the same size. There's no mechanism that makes a muscle more "toned" or "defined."

However, there *is* a simple two-step plan to make muscles *appear* more "toned" or "defined":

STEP 1. Make the muscles bigger.
STEP 2. Burn off the fat covering your muscles.

The *BFS* workout routines and nutritional guidance are designed to do both, with more emphasis on making muscles bigger in the Fall and Winter programs, shifting to a focus on burning fat in the Spring and Summer workouts. But rest assured: no part of my system ignores the basic facts of exercise science.

"I'm Trying to Build Size, Not Strength"

The human body isn't stupid. If it's going to overcome a genetic propensity toward low body weight, it needs a better excuse than "I just want to be bigger." Strength is the excuse. Give the muscles tasks that push their limits, using heavy weights and smart program design, and they'll get bigger to meet the increased need for strength.

In the fitness industry, someone who's just concerned with the aesthetics of muscles is said to be "all show and no go," which is really just a cutesy way of implying that they view their muscles as pure ornamentation and nothing more.

You could accuse me of advocating the same thing, given that the title of this book uses the words "built," "for," and "show," in that order. But I see no con-tradiction in acknowledging that all of us reading this want good-looking, eye-catching muscle, while telling you the best way to build it is to forget what your muscles look like and focus on what they can do.

You won't regret getting more "go" in pursuit of the "show." There's no downside to being as strong as you look, whether you demonstrate that strength by helping your friends move their furniture or by lifting an intimate friend onto a particular piece of furniture.

"I Do Curls Because I Want Big Arms"

All of us fall into the muscle-isolating trap, to some extent. But if you're a skinny guy, with a body that's reluctant to put on muscle mass, you may have the most to lose when you waste energy on isolation exercises.

Isolation exercises don't use a lot of muscle mass—an obvious point when you consider that the goal of an isolation exercise is to *not use* the muscles you aren't trying to isolate. But here's a not-so-obvious point: when you do a biceps curl or triceps extension, you aren't even recruiting the most important fibers within the muscles you're isolating. That's because you rarely use a lot of weight when you do those exercises. Your body's biggest, strongest muscle fibers, the ones with the most growth potential, simply don't come into play unless you're using heavy weights in low-repetition sets.

I can't recall ever seeing anyone do low-rep sets for their biceps and triceps, for one simple reason: as soon as you start lifting near-max weights, you can't even pretend to isolate muscles. You have to "cheat" by using less-strict movement patterns, which brings bigger muscles into the exercise.

Let's review:

- You can't build the biggest possible muscles unless you employ the biggest fibers within those muscles.
- To use those muscle fibers, you have to lift the heaviest possible weights.
- To lift the heaviest possible weights, you have to abandon the idea of isolating specific muscles, since your body will instinctively bring other, bigger muscles into the action.

So why bother trying to isolate? If you lift the heaviest possible weights during exercises that use the most muscle mass, you'll employ your body's biggest muscle fibers while doing the exercises safely and correctly.

THINGS FAT GUYS BELIEVE THAT KEEP THEM FAT

"If I Eat Before and After Workouts, My Body Won't Burn as Much Fat"

I'll get into nutrition much more in Part 3, but for now I'll leave it at this: skipping meals is the best way I know to *prevent* your body from using its stored fat for energy. Counterintuitive as it seems, regular meals, including pre- and postworkout nutrition, will promote steady fat loss. It works the same way whether you're lean or lardy. The more often you eat while you're doing a serious training program, the more fat you lose.

Your body needs fuel, pure and simple. A preworkout meal of protein and carbohydrates will actually enhance blood flow and help deliver nutrients to the muscles when they need it most: when you're breaking them down by working out. Similarly, a postworkout meal will help speed muscle growth and help you recover more quickly before your next formal (weight-lifting) or informal (woman-lifting) training session.

As you'll see when you get to Chapter 9, I'm a real hardass when it comes to postworkout nutrition. You have to have protein and carbs as soon as possible after lifting.

That said, I'm not particularly militant about preworkout meals. I don't think it's a good idea to work out on an empty stomach, so I tell my clients who like to work out in the morning that they should eat something first. What they eat, and how much they eat, is more of a personal thing. Later in the day, do what works best for you. If you can't train hard without eating something right before your workout, make sure you have something ready to eat. If you can get in a good workout two or three hours after your most recent meal, that's cool. I'm not going to tell you to ignore your body and follow some arbitrary guideline.

"I Need These Carbs for Energy So I Can Have Good Workouts"

Here's the flip side of the first belief: Some XXL lifters think they have to eat like skinny runners in order to get through their workouts. This means an abundance of carbohydrates in the form of food (bananas, bagels), drinks (Gatorade, Red Bull), and gels.

My rule: a guy with excess flesh should never *ever* eat or drink carbohydrates unless they're accompanied by protein. The combination of carbs and protein gives your muscles what they need to work and grow. Carbs by themselves provide energy that, in the absence of protein, can get stored as fat if it isn't needed for your workout.

You could say this is a contradiction of the point I made earlier about calories speeding up your metabolism. It's really not. Some types of calories speed up your metabolism more than others. Protein calories speed it up a lot; calories from carbs speed it up only a little.

I'm not a fan of working out on an empty stomach, as I said. So if you work out first thing in the morning, I think you really should eat something first, even if you aren't particularly hungry.

But at other times of day, use hunger and personal comfort as a guideline. I don't see the point in pumping excess preworkout calories into your body if you aren't hungry and are only doing it because you think you need the energy. As long as you've eaten something in the past couple of hours, and don't feel especially hungry, you have enough energy to work out.

Just make sure that whatever you eat has a mix of protein and carbs, and that you aren't adding more calories than you could hope to burn off in your workout.

"I Don't Need to Do Squats. I'm Already Big"

Right. And porn stars don't need to perform Kegel exercises, either.

A lot of guys are naturally big, and some of them put on muscle easily. I'm not one, and you probably aren't either, but we both know they're out there. Despite that fundamental difference, though, they still need to focus on the money-maker movements to get the results they want.

I've lost count of the number of wide-bodied guys I've come across who skip the big-muscle exercises and instead spend their time in the gym working their biceps, triceps, and deltoids. I understand the temptation; if you build muscle easily, you build it easily *everywhere*, including your arms and shoulders.

They forget that women will notice a big gut sooner than big guns. If you don't believe me, ask any woman you know if she's more turned *on* by nineteen-inch arms than she's turned *off* by a forty-inch waist.

The beauty of the moneymaker exercises is that they help anyone, no matter how thick or thin, develop a more athletic-looking physique. The process of building muscle speeds up your metabolism, and in the quest to whittle down your waistline, a faster metabolism is the best friend you can possibly have. Your shoulders get wider while your waist slims down, and you burn off some of the fat covering the muscles you want to show off.

"Everyone in My Family Is Fat. I'll Always Be Fat"

Unless every individual in your family does my workout programs and follows my dietary advice, and yet remains fat, I'm not accepting this argument.

HOW SKINNY-FAT GUYS END UP WITH THE WORST OF BOTH WORLDS

Some guys can have narrow shoulders, a sunken chest, and pipe-cleaner arms . . . and still carry excess flab around the middle. We call this "skinny-fat," and I wouldn't wish it on my worst enemies.

In my experience, a typical skinny-fat guy doesn't eat a lot of food. But what he does eat is suboptimal—"crap," in other words—and the way he eats it is even worse. He skips breakfast, then has fast food or Top Ramen for lunch and dinner. If you ask him how he spends his evenings, you'll get one of two answers: drinking beer with his friends until the single-digit hours, or posting on his blog until well past midnight. Or he might go drinking, come home, and spend the next hour or two posting his drunken thoughts. In any case, it's bad for his physique, bad for his health, and bad for online discourse.

There is some good news, however.

The skinny-fat guy can often make rapid progress when he commits himself to a good program, since his body will respond to just about any change in routine. Unlike the merely skinny guy, who might actually be in pretty good shape, or the big-bodied guy, who might be strong and have a lot of muscle beneath his fat, the skinny-fat guy is almost always severely undertrained.

But let's not kid ourselves: if you're skinny-fat, you need more than a good workout plan. Your diet probably sucks, too, and that's a direct consequence of your biggest problem: your lifestyle.

My friend and mentor Dan John has an amazing ability to break down complex psychological theories into simple and memorable sound bites. One of his favorites:

Your habits must match your goals.

Let's say your goal is to become a rodeo champion. Since you don't live on a ranch, you wouldn't stand a chance in the riding-and-roping categories. But you figure you have a fighting chance to become a champion bull rider. All it takes is balance, coordination, brass balls, and practice. Lots and lots and lots of practice. No matter how much you *look* like a cowboy, how much tobacco you can pack into your cheeks, or how many Waylon Jennings songs you know by heart, you won't get close to winning anything unless you put your ass on a hoofed animal as often as you possibly can.

But if the only moving creature you ride with any regularity is a mechanical bull at your local bar, and you only do that on Wednesdays in between rounds of karaoke, you can be pretty sure you won't need to worry about finding space for all those bull-riding trophies you hope to win.

Likewise, giving yourself a *BFS* body requires substantial changes to your daily routine.

YOUR OLD HABIT: *getting four to six hours of sleep per night, leaving you looking and performing like a cross between Ozzy Osbourne and Nick Nolte*

Despite what most of us think, the workouts you do in the gym don't build muscle. They *destroy* it. The point of a workout is to break down muscle tissue, which is subsequently rebuilt after you finish lifting. The better you manage that postworkout recovery, the better chance you have of emerging from your muscle-destroying experience with a stronger, leaner, and more muscular physique.

Just about everything you do in the hours and days following a muscle-damaging workout will affect your recovery, including sleep. A good night's sleep not only allows your body to continue the repair-and-rebuild process, but also gives your brain a chance to release hormones vital to that effort.

YOUR NEW HABIT: *a sleep schedule that allows for at least eight hours of sleep per night.*

Count backward from whenever you have to get up in the morning (or the following afternoon, if you're a college student). If you have to get up at 7 a.m., that means you have to be asleep by 11 p.m. the previous night. Note my choice of words: you're not just in bed by 11; you're in bed *and asleep.* Or, to get back to a reality-based prescription, you're in bed with your eyes closed, prepared to fall asleep.

That means that whatever reading or Web-surfing or TV-watching you feel compelled to do must be completed before 11. Every single electronic device in your room must be switched off before 11, even if it's just one minute before. Every light must be off. If the power strips on your TV or computer cast a glow, you might want to switch them off, too.

YOUR OLD HABIT: *eating just twice per day, and being asked "Do you want fries with that?" at least four times per week*

Two things I know for dead certain about guys: we hate being nagged, and we especially hate being nagged about food. If you're in college, or living the bachelor life, food seems a lot less important to you than it does to the naggers in your life. Your idea of a gourmet meal might be putting your microwave burrito on a plate instead of eating it right out of the plastic. As a guy who still heads over to Mom's house on weekends, I understand. Still, with a little practice, it's easy to keep a supply of healthy and tasty food on hand, and it's easy to learn to use that food in some quick and reliable meals. You don't have to channel your inner Emeril; you just have to follow some basic rules.

YOUR NEW HABIT: *eating at least three meals per day, preferably four to six meals and snacks*

The three-meal minimum starts with a solid breakfast no more than an hour after you wake up. Lunch and dinner will follow at sensible intervals. That is, if you eat breakfast at 8 a.m., you'll have lunch at 1 or 2 p.m., and dinner at 6 or 7. You don't want to have breakfast at 8, lunch at noon, and then dinner at 10:55 p.m., for reasons I explain in much more detail in Chapter 9.

It's also time to wean yourself off fast food. If you're eating out at fast-food joints three or more times per week, I want you to scale it down to one. When you do hit the drive-through—and, let's face it, all of us get into tight situations where there's no other alternative—skip the fries and order another burger instead. (That's a plain burger—meat and a bun. Leave the bacon, mayonnaise, and secret sauce for the tourists.) Quench your thirst with diet soda or water. These two changes alone could take an inch or more off your waist in less than a month.

YOUR OLD HABIT: *a workout "routine" that is anything but*

Without knowing you personally, I can make some assumptions about your workouts: either you don't have any regular routine—that is, if you work out at all, it's at random times, involving random exercises and techniques—or you have one that sucks. Based on my observations, that's how skinny-fat guys maintain their uniquely disadvantageous proportions.

YOUR NEW HABIT: *a workout routine that works for you*

Like everything else I've talked about so far in this section, this new habit requires a commitment. You have to decide that you're going to do a good workout routine (i.e., the *BFS* program), and you're going to do it at designated times on designated days. If you commit to a Monday-Wednesday-Friday training schedule, you're also going to commit to a specific hour on each of those three days. If you decide you're going to train after work, say from 6 to 7 p.m., then that hour on those three days is a permanent fixture on your calendar. It's no different from a meeting with your boss or an appointment with your parole officer. It's not optional.

I'll be honest with you: I can't sit here and predict exactly how fast you'll morph from what you look like now to what you want to look like. It might happen fast, it might be a struggle. But I *can* guarantee positive changes if you make this commitment. And I can just about guarantee mediocre results if you aren't consistent. The more often you show up, the faster your body will grow up.

YOUR OLD HABIT: *chronic time-wasting activities that sap your time and energy, and don't contribute to your health, wealth, or sex appeal*

I'm all for doing mindless things like watching a movie for the ninth time, surfing the Net for pictures of Jessica Biel, and posting my most superficial thoughts in online forums. I also love microbrews, and chances are good that you'll find me throwing a couple back with my buds on any given weekend.

But here's where my time-wasting habits probably differ from yours: I know when I'm screwing off—I recognize it for what it is—and I draw a firm line between what I allow myself to do in my leisure time and what I need to do the rest of my waking hours. In other words, I don't let the fun parts of my life prevent me from getting what I want in the serious parts.

I wasn't always this way. I used to assign a lot more value to useless, time-wasting activities—TWAs—some of which weren't even all that much fun. But then I realized something pretty simple, which gets back to the main theme of this section: My habits didn't match my goals. In some areas, my habits were preventing me from reaching my goals. They took time and energy, and they gave me . . . well, nothing.

Don't misconstrue what I'm saying: I'm entirely in favor of occasional debauchery—what's the point of being built for show if you don't take the new wheels out for a test-drive every now and then?—and I cherish the mindless activities I allow myself to do. If every minute of every day is devoted to reaching your goals, my guess is that you won't know what to do with yourself once you reach them.

The key is to identify and define your biggest TWAs, and decide which of them are worth what you invest in them.

YOUR NEW HABIT: *create a budget for your time-wasting or physique-impairing activities*

First you need a list of TWAs, and how much time and money (if any) you currently spend on each. Give each one a "relative satisfaction" score—an activity you absolutely enjoy the shit out of gets a 10, while something you could do without (harassing spammers, for example) gets a 1. Finally, take a guess at how much you could cut back on the activity before you started missing it.

TIME-WASTING ACTIVITIES				
Time-wasting activity	Hours wasted (per week)	Cost ($ per week)	Relative satisfaction (scale of 1–10)	How much you could cut back before you started missing it (0–100%)

Here's how a typical unmarried male might fill it out. Let's call him Tate, since he's a completely fictional character and bears no resemblance to anybody I know:

TIME-WASTING ACTIVITIES

Time-wasting activity	Hours wasted (per week)	Cost ($ per week)	Relative satisfaction (scale of 1–10)	How much you could cut back before you started missing it (0–100%)
Beers with friends	6	$25	10	0%
Watching *X-Men: The Last Stand* (or any other movie on DVD or cable) for the tenth time	2	$5	5	50%
Updating my blog	10	n/a	6	25%
Internet porn	7	n/a	Varies (depends on quality of porn)	–5%*
Chatting on the phone with people who dialed the wrong number	0.5	n/a	0	100%

* Negative value indicates Tate wouldn't mind increasing this particular TWA.

From this chart, it appears Tate could automatically gain four hours just by cutting back on his least satisfying TWAs. That, conveniently enough, gives him all the time he needs for the *BFS* workouts.

You'll notice that a lot of potential TWAs are missing from the list, including universal time-wasters like channel-surfing. I assume everyone reading this (not to mention the person writing it) wastes at least a little time each week flipping from channel to channel with no particular intent to watch any particular show. Here's my rule: you're allowed no more than five hours a week of unfocused TV watching or mindless Web surfing. And if it's a workout day, you are absolutely forbidden to channel-surf until after you've lifted.

Also, you'll notice that the "drinking with buds" category doesn't have a line to record the quantity of alcohol Tate consumes. That's because it, too, is subject to a blanket rule: you're allowed up to five drinks a week, but no more. You can have one drink a night with dinner, and spread your allocation over five nights, or have 'em all on Saturday night. As soon as you reach five, you must switch to water or another calorie-free beverage.

My point here, just to be 100 percent clear, is not that you need to turn into some kind of success-droid, spending every waking hour focused on your job or your bod. I just want you to be aware of how many things you waste time on that you don't enjoy all that much and wouldn't miss. Once you cut back on the least satisfying TWAs, you'll find you have a lot more time and energy for your workouts.

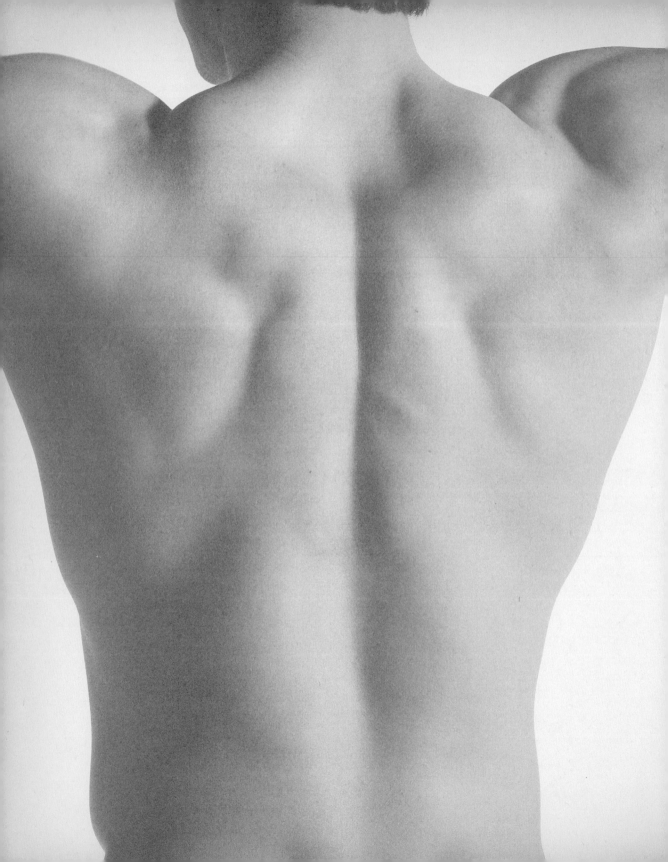

PART 2

Building the Head-Turning Body

CHAPTER FOUR

The Goods, and How to Get Them

I have a friend who played a few seasons in the NFL before an ankle injury forced him into early retirement. At five feet, ten inches and 190 pounds, Kris certainly looks like a football player: broad, muscular shoulders; a strong, flat midsection; and glutes that could probably crush walnuts. (Hey, shut up. *You* try spotting a guy when he's doing squats with more than five hundred pounds without noticing his ass.)

If you were to take the body of a running back and combine it with the strength of a lineman, you'd have a pretty good picture. On the football field, he was a relative shrimp, which helps explains why he was a placekicker. But in real life, walking among mortals like us, he's an Adonis.

I have it on good authority—in other words, he told me—that he pulled a fair number of women while he was in the league. It's no surprise that a pro athlete would get that kind of action. First, of course, is the fact that *he was a pro athlete.* It's like being in a rock band, only with muscles. Plus, he wasn't hurting for cash. When I asked him how much money he made, he said "minimum wage," which, since we're talking about the NFL, is not to be confused with "slave wage." (I don't know exactly what it was when he played, but if he had played his seventh season in 2007, league minimum would've been $595,000. That's not counting the dental plan.)

But here's the reason I'm telling you this: after his football career ended and he started his own home-appraising business, Kris still got laid. A lot. Why? Well, he's not ugly, but he's no Orlando Bloom, either. Financially, he's still doing okay, but it's nothing like his glory days. Does he brag about his status as a former pro? Actually, he's pretty humble in that area. He'll tell you if you ask, but he never brings it up unprompted. So how does a home appraiser inspire the same estrogenic frenzy he used to bring on as a stud athlete? How does he keep scoring years after he stepped off the field?

Simple. He stayed in shape. He maintained his athletic physique. He remained built for show.

But before I give you my definition of that term, let's back up and touch on something important that I've overlooked so far: What, exactly, makes a man attractive to a woman?

THE GOODS

David DeAngelo, author of *Double Your Dating* and all-around successful entrepreneur, has a terrific saying: "Attraction isn't a choice."

If you want proof, the next time you're out and about, just look around and count how many women you're instantly attracted to. You don't know a thing about them, other than what your eyes see. Do you think you made a conscious choice with any of this eye candy?

We guys are pretty simple when it comes to selecting a mate. See female, want female. If a woman is visually appealing, we'll probably be attracted to her. It's been biologically programmed into our genetic makeup, and it's not our choice.

(At least that's what we tell our girlfriends when we're caught looking at other females.)

But women are different. They have standards. They're constantly testing and judging you, often within the first ten seconds of interaction. They're looking for the telltale signs of just how good a baby-daddy you'll be, and how well you'll provide for the baby-mommy afterward.

Some of these signs are out of our control. You can't choose to be taller or to realign the symmetry of your ears, for example. (Chicks dig the good symmetry.) Income and "high social value" are also on their radar. So you'll be judged on what you're wearing, what you're driving, what you're drinking, and with whom you're doing it. A woman who's checking you out will also want some sign that you have an education comparable to hers. Granted, your academic achievements aren't easy to assess in the first ten seconds of visual contact, but it's safe to say that guys with Ivy League MBAs don't typically wear their ball caps sideways, show three inches of boxers above the top of their jeans, or hang out with guys who make fart jokes or share their World of Warcraft strategies in public places.

But let's assume a woman you've never met has scoped you out well enough to approve of your height, facial symmetry, and social status. She's decided you're not ugly, and probably aren't too stupid to hold a decent job. Remember, this is no more a choice for her than it is for you. Her subconscious brain has decided you're potentially okay.

Now we arrive at the part that's within your control, not to mention within my scope of expertise: your physique.

A strong, powerful body is a very positive indicator that you'll spawn children who'll grow up to be equally strong and powerful. If you build that body, you'll have an edge over the other guys she might be attracted to.

There's kind of a weird notion today that women are looking for Brad Pitt types—skinny dudes with ripped abs. (I should note, for the sake of pop-culture accuracy, that I'm talking about *Fight Club* Pitt, not the pumped-up Achilles Pitt we saw in *Troy.*) But a major study of singles' dating habits found that women prefer a guy with a body mass index around 27. That translates to two hundred pounds on a man who's six feet tall, which is approximately one and a third skinny Brad Pitts. It also, conveniently, is more or less the average size of a male adult in America today.

The important take-home lesson is this: Women aren't necessarily looking for a freak before they get their freak on. If all else is equal, a guy who's got The Goods should get the woman. So, what are The Goods?

Shoulders

A 2003 study in *Archives of Sexual Behavior* found that a proportion with shoulders about 40 percent wider than the waistline was rated most attractive by women. A 2006 study in the same journal found that the most sexually adventurous women preferred men with more masculine body types, which of course includes wide, athletic shoulders.

These aren't impossible standards. Far from it, really.

Any guy, no matter how big or slight he is when he starts training, can make his shoulders wider, relative to his waist, or narrow his waistline to make his shoulders look bigger. You don't have to be David Copperfield to create this visual magic. You just need to do workouts that are designed for that purpose.

Glutes

Show me a single, sexually active woman who says she doesn't care about the shape or size of a potential partner's backside, and I'll show you a woman who's lying.

Well-formed glutes, the kind that look like twin construction helmets, indicate sexual prowess and strength. Squats and deadlifts produce those glutes. A chair sitter's butt is the opposite of a weight lifter's. It's flat. I mean Kansas flat, with no break in the topography from shoulders to ankles. Nobody wants to sleep with a guy who reminds her of a mind-numbing drive along Interstate 70.

You'd think guys would figure this out, but I see no evidence of it. If anything, I see more guys walking around with I-70 butts, and fewer guys squatting and deadlifting. Few women I've met are looking for perfection, but I've never known one who wasn't turned off by a body that looks like a "before" picture on the bottom and an "after" picture on top.

Midsection

Notice I didn't say "abs." Guys of all ages are understandably obsessed with their six-packs. But getting that lean is difficult for most, and impossible for some. Maintaining high muscularity with low body fat is unrealistic for almost all of us. Even the cover models you see in fitness magazines, a genetically select group to begin with, need at least a week to diet down and dehydrate before they're ready for their close-ups. Sure, they look better than 99.9 percent of all humans even when they aren't in front of the cameras, but trust me when I say that nobody looks like he belongs on a magazine cover 365 days a year.

That's not to say you won't end up with ripped abs by the end of the *BFS* program. Some of you will. I just want to make it perfectly clear that abs like raviolis are a bonus, not a feature, of *Built for Show*.

What we're going to create here is a midsection that's athletic—flat, solid, and strong as hell. Like a football player's.

When you have The Goods from top to bottom—the shoulders, the midsection, the glutes—you'll finally have a body that looks the way male bodies are supposed to look, the way athletic beauty is portrayed in classic Greek and Roman sculpture. But more to the point, it's the way women want you to look.

But what about . . .

By now you've probably noticed what *isn't* on the list. The *BFS* programs don't put any special emphasis on pectorals, biceps, triceps, or calves. I know that what I just said is heresy, a thought crime in today's bar-body culture. But before you list your copy of *Built for Show* on eBay, let me explain:

All your muscles will grow in proportion to one another—your favorites and least favorites alike—when you do the basic strength exercises I include in *BFS*. Individual muscles rarely need any special attention.

Think back to Chapter 2 and the GTO-restoration analogy. You can't put the finishing touches on a body that hasn't yet been built. Moneymaker moves come first, polishing techniques later.

Which brings me to what is probably your most urgent question at this point in the narrative:

Are you telling me there aren't any freakin' curls in this program?

No, I'm not saying that. You'll find some in the Summer program, which is the last stage of the yearlong *BFS* training system. And you're welcome to start with that program, if you've already built a body that's almost ready for show, or if you really, really want to do some curls. But for all the reasons I just explained, they're a small part of the system. You'll understand why when you do the first three programs and realize that your arms have grown more without curls than they ever did with them.

CHAPTER FIVE

Before You Start the Workouts . . .

A guy's ideal physique shifts with the temperature. At least it does in Montana, where I live. We all want that summertime six-pack, but in the other three seasons, when most of us have to wear a shirt in public places, we want women to see that we offer more than a pretty face.

I've created four programs (Fall, Winter, Spring, Summer), with the goal of bringing out The Goods no matter the weather. Three of the programs take twelve weeks to complete, while the Winter program takes fourteen weeks. You can do the programs in the sequence they're presented, giving you a yearlong workout plan, or jump right into whichever one best suits your goals right now.

If you plan on doing it in order, starting with Fall and ending with Summer, you'll get what my fellow fitness geeks and I call a periodized workout program, which is the most sophisticated approach to strength training.

But before you jump into the programs, detailed in Chapter 7, let's look at some of the features of the system, especially some concepts and techniques that might be new to you.

Three Workouts per Week

I want you to work out three times a week on nonconsecutive days. If you aren't training at all right now . . . well, hell, that's three more workouts than you do in a typical week, which is certainly challenging enough. But for many of you, this is going to mean spending less time in the gym than you do now—a *lot* less, for those of you doing six-days-a-week routines you got from an old copy of *Ironman* you found in the dentist's office.

The motto here is "get in, work hard, get the hell out." If you can do that three times a week, you'll be able to make steady progress and achieve the gains you want. Frankly, there aren't many guys I've met who can handle more than three tough workouts a week without slacking off or piddling around with repetitive exercises and unnecessary sets and reps.

There's no dead space in these workouts. Almost every exercise hits multiple muscle groups and develops total-body strength and muscle size. If you work as hard as you should three days a week, you won't feel any urge to train more often.

Split Routines and Total-Body Training

The Fall and Winter programs feature what we call split routines. You'll work your upper body in one workout and your lower body in the next, and continue alternating throughout the programs. If you suffer from the KFC syndrome (big chest, chicken legs), this will take care of the problem. Your upper body and lower body will finally look like they belong to the same person.

The Spring and Summer programs shift to total-body workouts, meaning you work all your major muscles each time you hit the weight room. You'll develop strength and size proportionally, as you did in the Fall and Winter programs, but you'll also burn off more fat, thanks to the fact that you're doing serious lower-body exercises like squats or deadlifts three times a week. These workouts take more energy to do, and reward you with a bigger boost to your metabolism.

You'll also unleash more of your body's natural muscle-building hormones, which respond best to workouts that use the most overall muscle mass.

So why not do total-body workouts in all four seasons? Mainly because it's a lot harder to train this way. It helps to build a base of strength and conditioning first. The better shape you're in before you start the Spring and Summer programs, the faster you'll see fat melt away and the better your muscles will look as a reward for your hard work.

The Summer workouts also include some strategically placed "finishers" for eye-candy muscles like your biceps, triceps, and abs. I'm not a big fan of exercises that target specific muscle groups, as I've said thus far in *BFS,* but I'm happy to use them to add the final touches to a physique that's already lean and muscular.

Finally, you'll also do some intervals in the Summer program. These are short, intense cardio workouts in which you go hard for a specified period (sixty seconds, say), and then go slow for twice that amount of time as you recover. Done right, intervals attack the pockets of fat that somehow manage to hold out against the total-body weight workouts.

When you put it all together, you'll finish the Summer workouts with the leanest body possible for swimsuit season. Plus, you finally get to do curls.

Alternating Workouts

I already mentioned that you'll alternate upper- and lower-body workouts in the Fall and Winter programs. (In Winter, there are actually two for your upper body and two for your lower body, which I'll explain in Chapter 7.) Even when you do total-body workouts in Spring and Summer, you'll alternate two different workouts.

If you're new to lifting, or if you've never done formal routines like the ones in *BFS,* this can be a little confusing at first. But it's actually pretty simple. Workouts have their own names: A and B. (Feel free to marvel at my cleverness; I'll wait.) If you work out the way most of us do, following a Monday-Wednesday-Friday schedule, six weeks of training would look like this:

	Mon	Tues	Wed	Thurs	Fri	Sat	Sun
Week 1	A	Off	B	Off	A	Off	Off
Week 2	B	Off	A	Off	B	Off	Off
Week 3	A	Off	B	Off	A	Off	Off
Week 4	B	Off	A	Off	B	Off	Off
Week 5	A	Off	B	Off	A	Off	Off
Week 6	B	Off	A	Off	B	Off	Off

After six weeks, I'll change things up and give you new versions of A and B to do for the next six weeks. With equal cleverness, I call these six-week periods Phase 1 and Phase 2.

Alternating Sets

When you look at the workout charts in the next chapter, you'll notice that each exercise has a letter preceding it. The first exercise is either A or A1. If it's A1, the next exercise will be A2. The next pair of exercises will be designated B1 and B2. (Sometimes there's a B3, which might be followed by B4.)

If an exercise starts out with simply a letter (A), that means you do it in "straight sets"—you do the designated sets with the designated amount of rest following each of them.

If the exercises have a letter and a number (A1 and A2, for example) then you're going to do them in alternating sets. You do the first exercise (A1), rest for the designated time, do the second exercise (A2), rest for the designated time, and repeat until you've done all the required sets of both exercises.

Let's look at an example from the Fall program:

Exercise	Sets	Reps	Rest (seconds)
A1 Wide-grip cable row	4	8	60
A2 Dumbbell bench press	4	8	60

Translation:

Start with a set of eight wide-grip cable rows. Rest for sixty seconds. Do a set of eight dumbbell bench presses, and rest sixty seconds. Repeat the sequence (A1, rest, A2, rest) three more times before moving on to the next pair of exercises.

You'll note that this isn't a traditional "superset," in which you do two different exercises back-to-back without resting in between. My goal here is to give the muscles you're using in the first exercise more time to recover before you work them again. If it takes you twenty seconds to do a set of dumbbell bench presses, that means you have 140 seconds between the time you end one set of rows and begin the next one. Yes, you're doing another exercise in between, but you're using different muscles.

If you were doing straight sets of a single exercise, you'd have just sixty seconds to recover before you had to start the next set. Alternating sets allow more than twice the recovery time, which means you'll be able to work with heavier weights and make faster gains.

Varying Set-Rep Ranges

I could've made the workouts in *Built for Show* simple and easy to remember. I could've told you to do something like "three sets of twelve" or "five sets of five" for each exercise in each workout in each program, and then change things up across the board every few weeks.

But that's not the way I'd train myself or my clients, and it's not the way to get the fastest possible results.

So I'm going to use a system called "undulating periodization." The phrase itself is a crime against clarity, but the concept is easy to grasp: if you mix up the configuration of sets and reps from one workout to the next, your body will develop faster than it would if you only used one configuration for weeks or months at a time.

For example, in the first part of the Fall program, you'll use three different combinations of sets and reps: four sets of eight reps (4 x 8), five sets of five (5 x 5), and three sets of twelve (3 x 12). You'll always do 4 x 8 the first workout of the week, 5 x 5 the second workout, and 3 x 12 the third workout.

You already know that you're alternating the A and B workouts. So here's a repeat of the chart I used earlier to show you how a six-week schedule will look, this time adding the set-and-rep configurations you'll use each day:

	Mon	Tues	Wed	Thurs	Fri	Sat	Sun
Week 1	A (4 x 8)	Off	B (5 x 5)	Off	A (3 x 12)	Off	Off
Week 2	B (4 x 8)	Off	A (5 x 5)	Off	B (3 x 12)	Off	Off
Week 3	A (4 x 8)	Off	B (5 x 5)	Off	A (3 x 12)	Off	Off
Week 4	B (4 x 8)	Off	A (5 x 5)	Off	B (3 x 12)	Off	Off
Week 5	A (4 x 8)	Off	B (5 x 5)	Off	A (3 x 12)	Off	Off
Week 6	B (4 x 8)	Off	A (5 x 5)	Off	B (3 x 12)	Off	Off

As you can see, you're doing six distinct workouts in the first two weeks, without repeating any of them. The schedule starts over again in Week 3, and then again in Week 5. If you're training hard and eating right, you should be able to use heavier weights the second time through the schedule, and even heavier weights the third time.

I confess it would've been a lot simpler for you, and a lot easier for me, to skip this complication. But I think you'll make faster gains for three reasons:

First, you aren't developing one particular muscle quality at the expense of others. You aren't working only on pure strength (5 x 5), or muscle growth (4 x 8), or muscle endurance (3 x 12). All those qualities are important, so you'll develop all of them in the same program.

Second, you aren't hammering your joints into submission, as you would if you used relatively heavy weights and low reps (5 x 5) in every workout. And you aren't sacrificing strength and size gains by using relatively light weights and high reps (3 x 12) every time you go to the gym.

Finally, you aren't boring the shit out of yourself by doing something between (4 x 8) three times a week.

Rest and Recovery

Three types of recovery come into play during aggressive training programs like the ones in *BFS*:

REST PERIODS BETWEEN SETS AND/OR EXERCISES

As you saw earlier in this chapter, when I was explaining how to use alternating sets, I give you a specific amount of time to rest in between sets and exercises. These will vary from workout to workout, something that's very clear and easy to follow in the workout charts in Chapter 7. My method is pretty simple and intuitive: when you're using heavier weights (5 x 5), you'll have more time to recover between sets. And when you're using lighter weights (3 x 12), you'll have less.

On the days when you're having a really good workout, it'll seem like too much time in between sets, and you'll want to jump into the next one sooner than I suggest. On bad workout days (and we all have them), you'll feel as if you need more time to recover. Those decisions are up to you. I encourage you to stick to the prescribed rest times as much as possible, even if it means holding back on your best days and soldiering through on your worst. But I don't want to pretend I'm the Workout Police; no one will throw your ass out of the gym if you violate the rest codes. Do what you feel you need to do.

DAYS IN BETWEEN WORKOUTS

As I mentioned at the start of this chapter, three workouts a week is both your minimum and maximum. You'll always take one day off in between workouts, and sometimes you'll have two days. Don't e-mail me and ask if it's okay to do two workouts on back-to-back days. It's not. You always need at least one day in between to make sure your muscles, joints, and nervous system have the time they need to recover from one workout to the next.

Our natural tendency is to regard downtime as wasted time, thinking that if we aren't training, we aren't growing. The truth is the opposite: your muscles grow and your strength increases not when you're working out, but when you're *recovering* from a workout. Training itself is the stimulus, but the response comes during the period in between workouts. Cut it short, and you limit your gains.

REST WEEKS

Three of the *BFS* programs take twelve weeks to complete. The Winter program requires fourteen. Add them up, and you get fifty weeks of training. But sharp readers will remember that I promised a yearlong program. Speaking as a guy who had to take the same high school algebra class for three consecutive years before I finally passed it, even *my* math skills are strong enough to understand that a year is longer than fifty weeks. So what do you do with the extra weeks?

Nothing.

Seriously, I want you to take at least two full weeks off in a year of training. In fact, I'd like you to take a full week off after completing each program. That means the entire *BFS* program takes fifty-four weeks, or slightly more than a year. Here's why:

Different parts of your body recover at different speeds. Your connective tissues have a smaller blood supply than your muscles, so they usually lag behind in their development. Your bones have an even smaller blood supply, and they can use the extra recovery time as well. Finally, your nervous system can accumulate fatigue, a problem that could come back to haunt you down the road if you let it build up without relief. You might get burned out on training, or start losing sleep, or become more irritable than usual. (It's sort of like staying up all night to cram for finals. Do it too many nights in a row and before long you're such a dick that even your best friends won't pick up your calls before they go to voice mail.)

Trust me, you won't lose any of your hard-earned strength and size in a single week. In fact, you may actually find that you're bigger and stronger when you return to the gym, thanks to the time you took to allow your body to catch up on its recovery.

GETTING STARTED

You're almost ready to start. But before you do, I'm going to answer several questions before you think to ask them:

How do I warm up?

If you're like many guys, your idea of a warm-up is to jump on a treadmill for five minutes, walk or jog while you watch *Are You Smarter than a Fifth Grader?* on the little TV screen, and then jump right into your heaviest lifts. But even that is more of a warm-up than most guys with our demographic profile are willing to do.

A true warm-up involves four separate variables—physiological, hormonal, athletic, and technical. Lots of syllables there (plus a stupid acronym: PHAT), so let's break it down into language I don't have to stop to look up in a dictionary:

PHYSIOLOGICAL: Getting your body warm, as in raising your core temperature, is usually considered the goal of a warm-up. But it's actually just a byproduct of everything else. In other words, don't worry about whether you're actually hot and sweaty by the end of your warm-up. It'll happen on its own, and it's less important than the next three items on the list.

If you work out in the morning—in a cold garage or basement, for example—you probably want to devote a few minutes to a general warm-up. Five minutes or so on a stationary bike or treadmill is fine in that situation. At other times, particularly later in the day when your body temperature is naturally higher than it is first thing in the morning, you can skip that part.

HORMONAL: You want to get some adrenaline going. This is how your body prepares for serious physical activity, whether we're talking about a workout, a contest, a fight, or . . . you know, something else that's often life-changing and begins with an *f.* Like the first variable, it's something that happens if you're doing things right, as opposed to something you have to make happen, like the next two.

ATHLETIC: Lifting involves joint actions—bending and straightening. Each joint has an ideal range of motion. Before you start lifting, you have to make sure those joints are prepared to move through their ranges of motion, and to do so in a coordinated way.

I show you three good preworkout mobility drills in Chapter 6, which you should do before every weight workout. They're good to do on non-lifting days as well, but I mention that because only (a) it's true and (b) I wanted to give you a chance to laugh out loud at the idea of doing warm-up exercises when you aren't even planning to work out. It's like telling you to do your laundry before your clothes are dirty.

TECHNICAL: Now we get to the part where you actually practice the lifts you're going to do in your workout. There's no right or wrong way to do this, so I'll suggest some general guidelines that I use in my own workouts and that work well for my clients.

The key is to be prepared for the first exercise in your workout that day. How you warm up depends on how much weight you're going to use.

High reps, low weights: If you're going to do more than ten reps in your first set of your first exercise, or pair of exercises, you don't need an elaborate warm-up. You just have to make sure your body is ready for the specific range of motion required.

Let's say you're starting off with a single exercise like squats, using straight sets. The workout calls for three sets of twelve reps—3 x 12. A single warm-up set of six to eight reps is probably all you need. Use a weight that's about two-thirds of what you plan to use in your first set. In other words, if you think you'll use 135 pounds for twelve reps in your first set, warm up with ninety-five pounds.

If the workout calls for a pair of exercises to start—A1 and A2—then you want to do a warm-up set for each.

You probably don't need to do a warm-up set for the other exercises in that day's workout when you're using relatively light weights for high reps.

Medium reps, medium weight: When the workout calls for between six and ten reps per set, you want to do two warm-up sets of the first exercise or pair of exercises. Do the first warm-up set with about half the weight you plan to use in your first set, for five or six reps. Then do the second warm-up set with two-thirds of your first-set weight, and do three or four reps.

So if the first exercise is barbell bench presses, and you plan to use 135 pounds for eight reps in the first set, you could do five or six reps with sixty-five pounds for your first warm-up set, followed by three or four reps with ninety-five pounds.

After you finish the A exercise, or A1 and A2, you can decide if you want to do a warm-up set for each of the B exercises. It might help, and certainly wouldn't hurt.

Low reps, heavy weights: When you're doing fewer than five reps per set, I suggest three warm-up sets for your A exercise, or for both A exercises if you'll be alternating A1 and A2:

1. five reps with 50 percent of your first-set weight;
2. three reps with two-thirds of that weight;
3. one or two reps with 90 percent of your first-set weight.

If you're planning to use 185 pounds for the first set, you would use 95, 125 or 135, and 165 for your warm-ups. If you aren't a gym vet and don't understand why I use odd numbers in these examples, see the "Weights and Measures" sidebar (below) for an explanation.

For the B exercises, one or two warm-up sets should work.

Weights and Measures

If you're a weight-lifting novice, you may wonder why I use odd numbers like 95 and 135 pounds in these examples. Gym veterans will instantly understand that I use those numbers because they're easiest to apply with the equipment we use.

The Olympic barbell—the one you'll use for exercises like squats, deadlifts, and barbell bench presses—is seven feet long and weighs forty-five pounds. The most commonly used weight plates are ten, twenty-five, and/or forty-five pounds.

You'll also find five- and 2.5-pound plates, which come in handy when you're new to lifting. (Some gyms also have thirty-five-pound plates, which are about as useful as half-dollar coins.)

If you add a twenty-five-pound plate to each side of the forty-five-pound bar, you end up with ninety-five pounds. Put a forty-five-pound plate on each side and you have 135.

Other bars you might use weigh less. A standard barbell, for example, is usually six feet long and weighs ten pounds. This is the type of bar you'd typically find at a department store that sells weights, and it's the type many of us start off using in our basements or garages. It's easy to tell the difference between standard and Olympic plates: standard weight plates have a one-inch-wide hole in the middle; Olympic plates have a 2.5-inch hole. (Note: If you're thinking of buying a bench with uprights for bench presses, you have to choose one that's designed for the type of weights you're using. Benches designed for standard barbells aren't big or sturdy enough for Olympic weight sets. Standard barbells may or may not work with Olympic benches; it varies from bar to bar and bench to bench.)

An Olympic EZ-curl bar—the one with the zigzag in the middle that allows you to do curls with a diagonal grip, which is less stressful to your elbows and wrists than the underhand grip you'd use with a straight bar—weighs about twenty pounds.

Another device you'll see in most gyms is the Smith machine. This is a barbell on rails that many lifters will use for squats and bench presses. The bar looks like an Olympic barbell, but it only weighs fifteen pounds, rather than forty-five, which of course explains why it's so popular with the most ego-driven muscleheads. If you load it up with two forty-five-pound plates on each side, it looks like you're lifting 225 pounds, when in reality it's only 195.

Why is that important to lifters? Trust me, when you've been working out for a while with Olympic weights, you'll appreciate the ego boost that comes the first time you do a squat, deadlift, or bench press with two forty-five-pound plates on each side. On paper, a 225-pound bench press is just an incremental improvement over a 215-pound lift. But when you see those big plates on the bar, going from 215 to 225 feels like you've passed a test and finally arrived as a lifter.

Just don't deceive yourself into thinking that working with four plates on the Smith machine is the same thing. It's not even close. For that matter, it's best to avoid the temptation and avoid the Smith machine entirely.

How much weight should I use?

All the examples I just gave you are based on the idea that you know how much weight you'll use on that first set of each exercise. The more experience you have, the better you are at looking at a workout chart and guesstimating how much weight you can use for the most common exercises and the most common rep ranges.

It's particularly easy if you know or can guess how much weight you could lift for a single repetition of that exercise:

Number of reps	Percent of max	Weight you can expect to use with this percentage of your max*
1	100	225
2	95	215
4	90	200
6	85	190
8	80	180
10	75	170
12	67	155
15	65	145

* Assuming a one-rep max of 225 pounds, and rounded to the nearest five pounds.

The big flaw with this chart (which I borrowed from a textbook called *Essentials of Strength Training and Conditioning*) is that it assumes that the set in question is a one-time, all-out effort. But if the workout calls for 4 x 8, say, you aren't going to try to use 80 percent of your one-rep max on each set. Most of us would round down by a few percentage points—using 75 percent instead of 80, for example. That leaves a little something in the tank for the following sets, and acknowledges that we aren't capable of performing at our peak every single workout.

But let's be serious here: most of us have no idea what our max is on any lift. Even max bench presses went out of style before I picked up my first dumbbell. So we're all reduced to trial and error.

If you have some experience in the gym, and you're trying to figure out your starting weight for an exercise that's familiar to you (cable rows or dumbbell bench presses, for example), my advice is to go with your instinct, then deduct 25 percent. (Call it an excise tax for your ego.) Why? Because every double-testicled male I know—me, my friends, my clients, my clients' friends—will instinctively choose a weight that's too heavy. And the last thing you want to do is start out with a weight that's too heavy, forcing you to scale back in subsequent sets.

On the other hand, it's harmless to start out with a weight that's too light. If you really did undershoot your starting weight by 25 percent (if your instincts are reality-based, in other words), the worst that can happen is that you write off that set as an additional warm-up, then do your real first set with enough weight to get the desired effect.

But what is that desired effect? Well, that brings me to the next question.

Should I go to failure?

If it occurs to you to ask this question, you're probably an experienced lifter. For those with less time in the weight room, the question comes down to this: Should you go to the point at which you can't move the bar another inch? Should you stop before you get to that point? Or should you go to failure sometimes but not always?

I'll clear this one up fast: I don't advocate going to muscle failure on any of your sets.

Don't get me wrong; all of your sets should be challenging. They just don't need to go to the point at which your muscles are so weakened that your form is compromised. That's where injuries live, and I don't want you to even visit that neighborhood.

As a general rule, the last repetition of the last set of each exercise should be tough, but you should be able to complete it with good form. When you feel your form start to slip, or the speed of your repetitions slows down considerably, stop the set. You've done the work you need to do. Even if the workout chart says to do ten repetitions in that particular set, but you feel your form and rep speed start to change on the eighth rep, that's it. You've finished that set.

On earlier sets—the ones that precede the final set of an exercise—it's perfectly okay to get to the final repetition feeling as if you could do more. In fact, you probably want to finish the first set feeling as if you could've done two or even three more reps. If you get to the end feeling as if you haven't challenged your muscles, you can always increase the weight by the smallest possible increment for the second set. (Going from forty-five- to fifty-pound dumbbells, say.) If that doesn't work, bump the weight up again for your third set.

There's no one correct way to do my workouts, in terms of the weights you use. Some guys will use the same weight for every set (other than warm-ups, obviously). Others will want to increase the weight for every set. How the sets feel may even change from one workout to the next. One day you may not feel like you've really nailed an exercise until you get to the final set, but the next time you do that workout it could seem like your first and second sets were more productive than the third or fourth.

But this is a constant: you should never feel as if you weren't challenged just because you didn't go to absolute failure on one or more sets. This shit won't work if you don't work hard. You just don't have to work so hard on any one set that you fry your muscles and screw up the rest of your workout. There's no point in wasting it all on one set for the sake of ego or because you're trying to impress a woman. (They don't care how much you lift. It all looks heavy to them.)

How fast should I lift?

A lot of training programs you see these days tell you how fast to lift and lower weights on each repetition. The technical term is "tempo," and I can see both positive and negative aspects to paying attention to it. But when I tally them up, I think adhering to a trainer's idea of the perfect tempo for each rep is an unnecessary complication.

Some people naturally lift in a slow, controlled way, and others naturally jerk the weights around like they've got some place they'd rather be. Trying to get everyone moving at the same speed makes it feel unnatural for everybody. This isn't synchronized swimming we're talking about here.

So let's make it easy: I want you to lower the weight in a controlled manner, and lift it as fast as possible while maintaining good form. I don't want you taking six or eight or fifteen seconds to perform one rep (believe it: some trainers really tell you to lift that way), and I certainly don't want it to look like you're having a seizure.

Whatever allows you to work hard with good form is probably okay.

Do I have to keep a training log?

Yes. It's absolutely nonnegotiable. I know what you may be thinking: "I'm going to look stupid carrying a clipboard around." Too damn bad.

Take a look around the gym and you'll see two types of people who carry training logs—beginners and serious, advanced lifters. You may be starting off as the first, but if you keep a training log that details the weight you used, how you feel, and how much progress you've made, you'll quickly become one of the latter and leave the poseurs and frat boys flexing their biceps in the mirror in your dust.

You can either photocopy the blank chart (page 63) or go to builtforshow .com and download a copy for yourself.

BUILT FOR SHOW

SEASON/PHASE:

WORKOUT:

Exercise	Sets	Reps	Set 1	Set 2	Set 3	Set 4	Set 5	Set 6	Rest
Workout									
Workout									
Workout									
Workout									
Workout									
Workout									
Workout									
Workout									
Workout									
Workout									
Workout									
Workout									
Workout									
Workout									
Workout									
Workout									
Notes:									

HOW TO USE THE LOG

I'll once again use an example of alternating sets from the Fall program, Phase 1. You'll do the 4 x 8 configuration three times in the six-week phase. You chart each set by noting the weight you use, followed by a slash, followed by the number of reps you complete with that weight. Here's how your workouts might go, and how you'd chart them:

BUILT FOR SHOW

SEASON/PHASE: *FALL, Phase 1*

WORKOUT: *A*

Exercise	Sets	Reps	Set 1	Set 2	Set 3	Set 4	Set 5	Set 6	Rest
A1 Wide-grip cable row	*4*	*8*							*60*
Workout 1			*40/8*	*45/8*	*50/7*	*50/6*			
Workout 4			*50/8*	*50/8*	*50/8*	*50/7*			
Workout 7			*50/8*	*55/8*	*55/7*	*55/5*			
Workout									
Workout									
A2 Dumbbell bench press	*4*	*8*							*60*
Workout 1			*35/8*	*40/8*	*45/7*	*45/5*			
Workout 4			*40/8*	*45/8*	*45/8*	*45/7*			
Workout 7			*45/8*	*50/7*	*50/6*	*50/5*			
Workout									
Workout									

The first thing you'll notice here is that you didn't get exactly eight reps in each set. Sometimes you fall short of that. When you do, it's no problem; just start with that weight the next time you do that combination of sets and reps. When you easily get eight reps with that weight on every set, or almost every set, you're ready to move up to a heavier weight. And you always want to challenge yourself more the last time you do any workout in any phase—that's the time to get more aggressive, even if it means falling a couple reps short of the target.

CHAPTER SIX

Unlocking the Goods

I consider strength training an athletic activity. While it does make you look more athletic and make you better at sports, it's important to note that training itself is athletic. If you do it without preparing your body, you'll get hurt, same as the guy who plays touch football one spring day after a winter on his couch, and pulls a hamstring when he tries to run a deep pass route.

The mobility exercises in this chapter should be done as part of your warm-up. I give them their own chapter because I want to emphasize their importance beyond their value as warm-up exercises, for these reasons:

MOBILITY MAKES YOU A BETTER LIFTER

If your mobility is limited or unbalanced—if you're tighter on one side than the other—your strength will also be limited or unbalanced. You might also have compromised form on key exercises, like squats.

MOBILITY HELPS YOU STAY HEALTHY ENOUGH TO LIFT

A guy with suboptimal joint mobility is more likely to hurt himself in the weight room. Two of these three exercises focus on the hip joints, and with good reason: tight hips can lead to joint injuries above or below—bum knees, a bad back, or even a tweaked shoulder, as I explain in a moment.

MOBILITY MAKES YOU BETTER IN BED

You can't be a bedroom Baryshnikov if you move like you just got released from a full-body cast. The basic pelvic thrusting isn't particularly complex, as human movements go, but overly tight muscles and connective tissues can make your maneuvers less graceful than your partner would like them to be. The better you're able to move, the better the result.

MOBILITY SAVES YOUR SHOULDERS

According to my friend Bill Hartman, a physical therapist and trainer in Indianapolis whose knowledge of human movement borders on genius, a guy with tight hips is very likely to end up with shoulder problems. The full explanation requires a half-hour PowerPoint presentation, but here's the short version:

Imagine that all your muscles and connective tissues are a highway system. Everything connects to something else, and the roads don't end until they hit the terminal points of your body—your fingers, toes, and skull. Some parts of your body act as intersections, and some act like hubs. Your hip joints are hubs; lots of connective-tissue paths converge here and then radiate out to new destinations. Your shoulder blades are intersections, places where several paths crisscross. If something goes wrong in the hub, it's going to affect the intersections farther along the trail. That's why a problem in your left hip—tightness, weakness, injury—might lead to an injury in your right shoulder.

TERM LIMITS: THE DIFFERENCE BETWEEN MOBILITY AND FLEXIBILITY

Mobility refers to the range of motion of joints. *Flexibility* refers to the length and range of motion of muscles. When you hold a stretch for a specific amount of time, your goal is to improve flexibility. In other words, you're trying to lengthen the muscle. When you do mobility exercises, your focus is on joints—making sure they'll allow the specific movements you need to do in your upcoming workout.

Why wouldn't they? Sometimes the connective tissues on one side of a joint get shorter, weaker, or tighter than they should be, due to injury, inactivity, or the way you use that particular part of your body over a long period of time. If you're right-handed, for example, you're naturally going to use your right arm and leg differently from the way you use your left arm and leg, so over time you'll develop imbalances.

Flexibility exercises can be useful, as long as you do them after a strength workout, or on separate days. (The consensus today is that you shouldn't do them before, since they might compromise your strength and power.) But mobility exercises are more important, since mobility is more directly connected to performance and injury prevention.

The exercises

Set aside five minutes before your weight workout to do the following sequence of exercises. For the sake of simplicity, I describe the exercises as you see them in the photos. Sometimes I start with my right leg, sometimes with my left. You, on the other hand, should always start with your weaker or nondominant side—usually your left if you're right-handed.

Leg swings

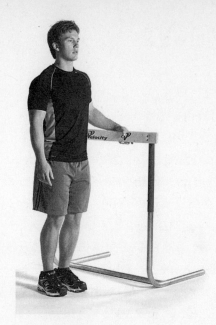

Stand with your left side two to three feet away from a wall or something similarly sturdy. Put your left hand on the wall at waist height. You want your feet hip-width apart, toes pointing forward. Now swing your right leg forward and back, keeping it straight but not locked at the knee or ankle. You aren't kicking here; you don't want to put any power behind the swings. You just want your leg to move freely. Do ten swings, then switch sides and repeat with your left leg.

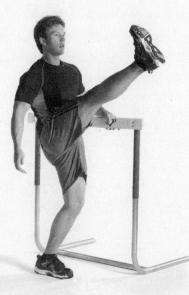

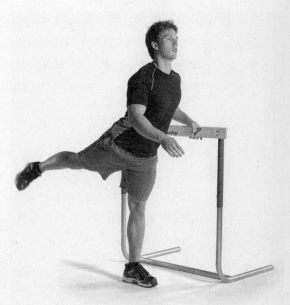

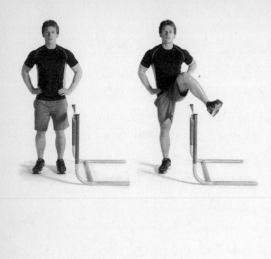

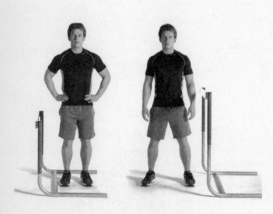

Lateral over-under drill

This is an exercise I picked up from my friend Robert dos Remedios, author of *Men's Health Power Training*.

Stand with your feet shoulder-width apart, toes pointing forward, and knees bent slightly. Keeping your shoulders square, imagine that you're stepping laterally (to the side) over a hurdle that's about the height of your middle thigh. Step over with your left leg, then over with your right. Now, with your feet once again shoulder-width apart, sink down into a deep squat, keeping your heels flat on the ground, and imagine stepping with your left leg first underneath a second hurdle that's about hip height.

After you clear the imaginary hurdle, stand up, with your feet once again shoulder-width apart. Now you're going to do the exercise in reverse: squat down, and go under the imaginary hurdle with your right leg first. Stand up after you clear the hurdle, and step over the other imaginary hurdle with your right leg, then your left.

That's one repetition. Do a total of three.

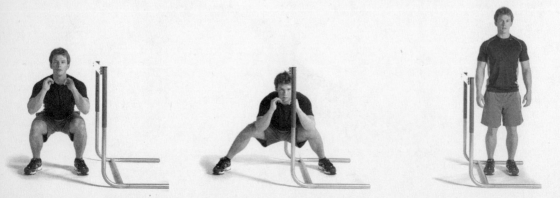

T push-up

Get into push-up position, with your arms straight down from your shoulders, your feet together, and your weight resting on your palms and toes. Your body should form a straight line from your neck to your ankles.

Bend at the elbows and lower your chest until it's two or three inches from the floor. Push back up, but as you do lift your right hand off the floor and rotate your shoulders to the right. Your eyes should follow your right arm throughout the movement. Finish with your right arm pointing straight up to the ceiling, with your torso and hips rotated 90 degrees from the starting position. Your arms and body should form a *T.* Hold that position for two seconds.

Reverse the movement so you're back in the starting position for a push-up. Immediately do another push-up, this time lifting your left arm and rotating to your left side. Again, hold that position for two seconds.

That's one repetition. Do a total of four reps—that is, four T push-ups to each side.

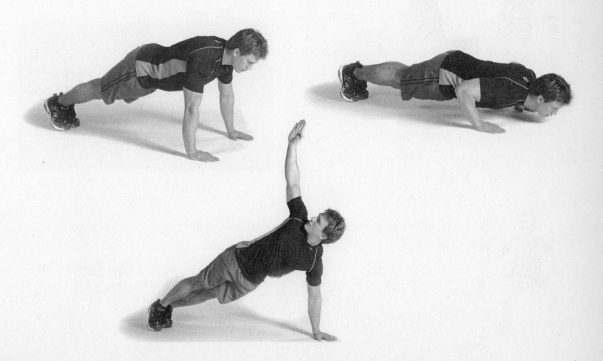

CHAPTER SEVEN

The *Built for Show* Programs

Now that you know what you need to know to do these workouts, it's time to plunge in, put some calluses on your palms, and build some of that muscle you've been promised since the opening pages of this book.

FALL

The Fall workout is designed to make muscles bigger, using fairly simple exercises and slightly more complex training techniques.

I've already explained how to do alternating sets, so you know what you're supposed to do when you see A1 and A2, or B1 and B2, on the workout charts. But you'll notice in Workout A that the C1 and C2 exercises require a different number of sets—two for the C1 exercise (reverse crunches) and one for C2 (the plank). It's not a typo. I want you to do the first set of reverse crunches, rest thirty seconds, do the plank as described, rest thirty seconds, then do the second and final set of reverse crunches.

You'll also notice something different going on in the B workout.

The first two exercises—front squats (A1) and step-ups (A2)—use the same rotating system of sets and reps that you employ throughout the A workout. But the next two exercises—B1 and B2—use a different, more straightforward type of progression. You'll do one set of each exercise the first two weeks of the Fall program, then add a set for the third and fourth weeks, then add a third set for the final two weeks.

I did it that way because those exercises involve a bit of a learning curve to get right. Rather than have you do a lot of sets before you get a feel for the exercises, which might get your body locked in on the wrong technique, you'll gradually increase the sets and reps. That way, your training volume increases along with your competence in the exercises.

These explanations and instructions apply to the workouts in Phase 2 as well as those in Phase 1, even though you'll be starting out with a slightly more challenging workload in Phase 2.

Phase 1

WORKOUT A (UPPER BODY)			
Exercise	Sets	Reps	Rest (seconds)
A1 Wide-grip cable row			
Workouts 1, 4, 7	4	8	60
Workouts 2, 5, 8	5	5	90
Workouts 3, 6, 9	3	12	45

continued on next page

Exercise	Sets	Reps	Rest (seconds)
A2 Dumbbell bench press			
Workouts 1, 4, 7	4	8	60
Workouts 2, 5, 8	5	5	90
Workouts 3, 6, 9	3	12	45
B1 Chin-up or underhand-grip lat pulldown			
Workouts 1, 4, 7	4	8	60
Workouts 2, 5, 8	5	5	90
Workouts 3, 6, 9	3	12	45
B2 Dumbbell shoulder press (neutral grip)			
Workouts 1, 4, 7	4	8	60
Workouts 2, 5, 8	5	5	90
Workouts 3, 6, 9	3	12	45
C1 Reverse crunch	2	15	30
C2 Plank	1	1*	30

* Hold for 60 seconds. If you can't hold for the entire 60 seconds, hold as long as you can, rest for that exact amount of time, then repeat until you reach a total of 60 seconds in the plank position.

WORKOUT B (LOWER BODY)			
Exercise	**Sets**	**Reps**	**Rest (seconds)**
A1 Front squat			
Workouts 1, 4, 7	4	8	60
Workouts 2, 5, 8	5	5	90
Workouts 3, 6, 9	3	12	45
A2 Step-up			
Workouts 1, 4, 7	4	8**	60
Workouts 2, 5, 8	5	5	90
Workouts 3, 6, 9	3	12	45

continued on next page

Exercise	Sets	Reps	Rest (seconds)
B1 Supine hip extension/leg curl			
Workouts 1, 2, 3	1	4–8	30
Workouts 4, 5, 6	2	6–10	30
Workouts 7, 8, 9	3	8–10	30
B2 Cable wood chop			
Workouts 1, 2, 3	1	8–10**	30
Workouts 4, 5, 6	2	8–10	30
Workouts 7, 8, 9	3	8–10	30
C Side plank	1	1*	n/a

* Hold for 30 seconds on each side. Don't rest as you switch from one side to the other. If you can't hold for the entire 30 seconds, hold as long as you can, rest for that exact amount of time, then repeat until you reach a total of 30 seconds in the side-plank position. Then switch sides and repeat.

** Each side. Start each set with your weaker or nondominant side—probably your left if you're right-handed.

Phase 2

WORKOUT A (UPPER BODY)			
Exercise	Sets	Reps	Rest (seconds)
A1 Barbell bent-over row (underhand grip)			
Workouts 1, 4, 7	6	5	90
Workouts 2, 5, 8	4	10	60
Workouts 3, 6, 9	3	15	45
A2 Dumbbell incline bench press			
Workouts 1, 4, 7	6	5	90
Workouts 2, 5, 8	4	10	60
Workouts 3, 6, 9	3	15	45

continued on next page

Exercise	Sets	Reps	Rest (seconds)
B1 Wide-grip lat pulldown			
Workouts 1, 4, 7	6	5	90
Workouts 2, 5, 8	4	10	60
Workouts 3, 6, 9	3	15	45
B2 Dip			
Workouts 1, 4, 7	6	5	90
Workouts 2, 5, 8	4	10	60
Workouts 3, 6, 9	3	15	45
C1 Reverse crunch	3	15	30
C2 Side plank	2	1*	30

* Hold for 30 seconds on each side. Don't rest as you switch from one side to the other. A set is a 30-second hold on each side. (By this point, you should be able to hold for the full 30 seconds.)

WORKOUT B (LOWER BODY)			
Exercise	Sets	Reps	Rest (seconds)
A1 Deadlift			
Workouts 1, 4, 7	4	8	60
Workouts 2, 5, 8	5	5	90
Workouts 3, 6, 9	3	12	45
A2 Bulgarian split squat			
Workouts 1, 4, 7	4	8**	60
Workouts 2, 5, 8	5	5	90
Workouts 3, 6, 9	3	12	45
B1 Goblet squat			
Workouts 1, 2, 3	2	4–6	30
Workouts 4, 5, 6	2	6–8	30
Workouts 7, 8, 9	3	6–8	30

continued on next page

Exercise	Sets	Reps	Rest (seconds)
B2 Cable reverse wood chop			
Workouts 1, 2, 3	2	8–10**	30
Workouts 4, 5, 6	2	8–10	30
Workouts 7, 8, 9	3	8–10	30
C Plank	2	1*	60

* Hold for 60 seconds, rest 60 seconds, then repeat. By this point you should be able to hold a plank for 60 seconds in the first set. If you can't hold for the entire 60 seconds in the second set, hold as long as you can, rest for that exact amount of time, then repeat until you reach a total of 60 seconds in the plank position.

** Each side. Start each set with your weaker or nondominant side—probably your left if you're right-handed.

WINTER

Muscle strength is the key to muscle growth, which is why this program pushes you to work with progressively heavier weights in the classic strength-building exercises.

The biggest change you'll see in the Winter program is the most superficial: instead of alternating A and B workouts, each of which you do nine times in six weeks, you'll have A, B, C, and D workouts, and do each five times. Because there are more total workouts per phase, you'll need fourteen weeks to complete the Winter program, rather than twelve.

Now let's talk about the important differences. In Phase 1, the workouts open with an unusual combination of sets and reps. You'll do three sets of four reps, then finish with a set of ten—what we commonly call a "back-off set," for reasons I explain in a moment.

You'll want to do three warm-up sets before that first exercise, as I described in Chapter 5. When the workout starts with A1 and A2 exercises, do three warm-ups for each exercise. Your first set of four reps should be challenging—the weight should be heavy, possibly heavier than anything you used in the entire Fall program for the same exercise. Then you want to use more on the second set of four, and still more on the third. You still want to be able to complete all four reps, but it's okay if you fall short.

As I said in Chapter 5, there's an art to choosing weights for workouts like this, and sometimes you choose a little too much. You just don't want to choose weights that are *way* too much, so you barely complete one or two reps on that final set of four. This isn't powerlifting. It's strength training, with an emphasis on *training*. You're training your muscles to be stronger, not testing their strength.

That said, you also don't want to undershoot, starting out with weights that are so light that by the third set you still get all four reps easily.

About that back-off set: since it calls for ten reps, instead of four, you'll have to use a much lighter weight. And since it comes after three low-rep sets in which you used progressively heavier weights, you'll probably have to use a lighter weight than you'd ordinarily use for a set of ten. I'll tell you this up front: you probably won't choose an appropriate weight for that back-off set the first time you try it. It's okay to mess up. Consider that first attempt an experiment, and try to get closer to the right weight the next time you do that workout. The goal is to use a weight that allows you to do ten reps with some effort, but not one that forces you to go to complete muscle failure.

Once you get past those A exercises, you'll use several different set-rep combinations. Sometimes you'll do three sets of eight, which you can do with the same weight on each set (if you happen to pick the appropriate weight for the first set), or with more weight on each set. Sometimes you'll do two sets of four, followed by a back-off set of ten reps. In that case, try to use more weight on the second set of four.

That's what you need to know for Phase 1. Phase 2 offers an entirely new technique, called "wave loading." You'll use two different types of wave loading.

The first type of wave loading employs six sets. The reps go like this: five, four, two, five, four, two. Even though it looks like one of those questions from an online IQ test—"identify the next number in the sequence . . . unless you're not as smart as you *think* you are"—it's really a cool way to use progressively heavier weights with lower reps. You'll start the first wave with a set of five reps. Increase the weight and do a set of four reps. Increase the weight yet again and do two reps. Easy enough, right? But now you're going to do a second wave, this time using more weight on the sets of five, four, and two reps.

Here's how it might work for any given exercise:

Set	Reps	Weight used
1	5	150
2	4	160
3	2	170
4	5	155
5	4	165
6	2	175

The first time through these workouts, don't push yourself to set personal records. Just get used to the technique. Then get more aggressive the second, third, and fourth times you do this type of wave loading. By the fifth and final workout, you should be using weights that you couldn't have imagined using at the start of the program. Just make sure you use a spotter when you bench press with weights this close to your maximum.

On squats, set up the safety rails of a squat rack so you can easily escape if you find yourself stuck in the bottom position with a heavy barbell on your shoulders. You can also use a spotter, who would stand behind you, and help you complete your final rep if you get stuck midway.

The rest of the exercises are perfectly safe to do without a spotter.

The second type of wave loading uses four sets, with these reps: four, six, four, ten. Use slightly less weight for the set of six than you did for the first set of four, and use heavier weights on the second set of four than you used on the first. Then finish with the back-off set of ten reps.

Phase 1

WORKOUT A (LOWER BODY)			
Exercise	Sets	Reps	Rest (seconds)
A Squat	4		120
Set 1		4	
Set 2		4	
Set 3		4	
Set 4		10	
B1 Dumbbell Romanian deadlift	3	8	60
B2 Reverse lunge	3	8**	60
C Reverse crunch	3	15	30

** Each leg. Start with your weaker or nondominant side—probably your left if you're right-handed.

WORKOUT B (UPPER BODY)			
Exercise	Sets	Reps	Rest (seconds)
A1 Barbell bent-over row	4		120
Set 1		4	
Set 2		4	
Set 3		4	
Set 4		10	
A2 Barbell incline bench press	4		120
Set 1		4	
Set 2		4	
Set 3		4	
Set 4		10	

continued on next page

Exercise	Sets	Reps	Rest (seconds)
B1 Dumbbell shoulder press	3		60
Set 1		4	
Set 2		4	
Set 3		10	
B2 Wide-grip lat pulldown	3		60
Set 1		4	
Set 2		4	
Set 3		10	
C Plank	3	1*	60

* Hold for 60 seconds, rest 60 seconds, then repeat two more times. By this point you should be able to hold a plank for 60 seconds in the first two sets. If you can't hold for the entire 60 seconds in the third set, hold as long as you can, rest for that exact amount of time, then repeat until you reach a total of 60 seconds in the plank position.

WORKOUT C (LOWER BODY)			
Exercise	Sets	Reps	Rest (seconds)
A Deadlift	4		120
Set 1		4	
Set 2		4	
Set 3		4	
Set 4		10	
B1 Bulgarian split squat	3	8**	60
B2 Supine hip extension/leg curl	3	8–12***	60
C Swiss-ball crunch	3	8	30

**Each leg. Start with your weaker or nondominant side—probably your left if you're right-handed.

*** If you can easily get ten or more reps with good form, progress to the one-leg ("Level 3") version of the exercise (shown on page 119). If you're stuck in between—you can get ten with two legs, but can't do very many with one leg, or you can do the unilateral version with one leg but not the other—then do the two-legged version with more reps.

WORKOUT D (UPPER BODY)			
Exercise	Sets	Reps	Rest (seconds)
A1 Chin-up	4		120
Set 1		4	
Set 2		4	
Set 3		4	
Set 4		10^	
A2 Barbell push press	4		120
Set 1		4	
Set 2		4	
Set 3		4	
Set 4		10	
B1 Wide-grip cable row	3		60
Set 1		4	
Set 2		4	
Set 3		10	
B2 Dumbbell bench press	3		60
Set 1		4	
Set 2		4	
Set 3		10	
C Side plank	2	1*	45

* Hold for 45 seconds on each side. Don't rest as you switch from one side to the other. A set is a 45-second hold on each side. By this point, you should be able to hold for the full 45 seconds on the first set. If you can't hold that long on the second set, hold as long as you can, rest for that exact amount of time, then repeat until you reach a total of 45 seconds in the side-plank position.

^ You'll probably need to do underhand-grip lat pulldowns instead of chin-ups for this set of ten. (If you can't do any chin-ups, even for the sets of four, use an assist machine or do underhand-grip lat pulldowns instead.)

Phase 2

WORKOUT A (LOWER BODY)			
Exercise	**Sets**	**Reps**	**Rest (seconds)**
A Squat	6		120
Set 1		5	
Set 2		4	
Set 3		2	
Set 4		5	
Set 5		4	
Set 6		2	
B1 Dumbbell Romanian deadlift	4		60
Set 1		4	
Set 2		6	
Set 3		4	
Set 4		12	
B2 Reverse lunge	4		60
Set 1		4**	
Set 2		6	
Set 3		4	
Set 4		12	
C Reverse crunch	3	12	30

**Each leg. Start with your weaker or nondominant side—probably your left if you're right-handed.

WORKOUT B (UPPER BODY)			
Exercise	Sets	Reps	Rest (seconds)
A Barbell incline bench press	6		120
Set 1		5	
Set 2		4	
Set 3		2	
Set 4		5	
Set 5		4	
Set 6		2	
B1 Barbell bent-over row	4		60
Set 1		4	
Set 2		6	
Set 3		4	
Set 4		12	
B2 Dumbbell shoulder press	4		60
Set 1		4	
Set 2		6	
Set 3		4	
Set 4		12	
B3 Wide-grip lat pulldown	4		60
Set 1		4	
Set 2		6	
Set 3		4	
Set 4		12	
C Plank	2	1*	60

* Hold for 75 seconds, rest 60 seconds, then repeat.

WORKOUT C (LOWER BODY)			
Exercise	**Sets**	**Reps**	**Rest (seconds)**
A Deadlift	6		120
Set 1		5	
Set 2		4	
Set 3		2	
Set 4		5	
Set 5		4	
Set 6		2	
B1 Supine hip extension/leg curl	4		60
Set 1		4***	
Set 2		4	
Set 3		4	
Set 4		12	
B2 Bulgarian split squat	3		60
Set 1		4**	
Set 2		6	
Set 3		4	
Set 4		12	
C Swiss-ball crunch	2	15	30

** Each leg. Start with your weaker or nondominant side—probably your left if you're right-handed.

*** Do the hardest version of the exercise for the four-rep sets, and then switch to an easier version for twelve reps in the final set.

WORKOUT D (UPPER BODY)			
Exercise	Sets	Reps	Rest (seconds)
A Chin-up	6		120
Set 1		5	
Set 2		4	
Set 3		2	
Set 4		5	
Set 5		4	
Set 6		2	
B1 Barbell push press	4		60
Set 1		4	
Set 2		6	
Set 3		4	
Set 4		12	
B2 Cable row	4		60
Set 1		4	
Set 2		6	
Set 3		4	
Set 4		12	
C Side plank	3	1*	45

* Hold for 45 seconds on each side. Don't rest as you switch from one side to the other. A set is a 45-second hold on each side, followed by 45 seconds of rest.

SPRING

I've been emphasizing the importance of an athletic look throughout *BFS*. That is, *looking like an athlete*. On the one hand, anyone with above-average strength and muscle mass will probably look more athletic than a guy with the same type of frame who's weaker and less muscular. But the women don't necessarily go wild over the guys with the *most* strength and muscle mass. You don't find a lot of smokin'-hot babes hanging out at powerlifting contests, but you can't turn around at a beach volleyball tournament without bumping into two of them. And if you've ever been to a professional bodybuilding show, you know there's a particular type of woman who hangs out there, and it's not a type you could easily describe with the nouns and adjectives you learned in school.

The difference between the two venues—other than the fact that volleyball takes place on a sunny beach and bodybuilding involves human beings covered in barbecue sauce to give the *illusion* that they've spent time on a sunny beach—is that the guys playing in the sand look like athletes. They aren't shredded like the bodybuilders, they aren't as strong as the powerlifters, and they don't have a fraction of the muscle mass of either group, but they look like guys who know how to use what they have. Or, put another way, they only have what they can use.

So this is the part of the program where we start honing your body into one that's leaner, faster, more powerful, and more athletic. You'll continue to develop strength and muscle mass, but you'll also shift from split routines to total-body workouts, which (as I warned in Chapter 5) are harder to do, and which improve your overall conditioning while giving whatever fat you have fewer reasons to hang around.

Part of that fat-shedding stimulation comes from new exercises like dumbbell snatches, barbell clean pulls, jump squats, and jump lunges. They're more challenging, so they help you increase your speed, power, and coordination. Which brings me to an important programming note: the power exercises use a different type of progression than the others. You'll start with three sets of five reps the first three times you do that particular workout, then go to 4 x 4 for the next three workouts, and finish with 5 x 3. The goal is to give you some time to master the exercises before you start working with heavier weights and lower reps.

Getting back to my original point in this introduction to the Spring programs, it's time to add some finesse to your bigger, stronger body, now that you've shed your winter coat. The changes might be subtle at this point, but if someone's looking closely enough, she'll notice.

Phase 1

WORKOUT A (TOTAL BODY)			
Exercise	Sets	Reps	Rest (seconds)
A Dumbbell snatch			
Workouts 1, 2, 3	3	5**	75
Workouts 4, 5, 6	4	4	75
Workouts 7, 8, 9	5	3	75
B1 Front squat			
Workouts 1, 4, 7	2	20	45
Workouts 2, 5, 8	5	5	90
Workouts 3, 6, 9	4	10	60
B2 Step-up			
Workouts 1, 4, 7	2	20**	45
Workouts 2, 5, 8	5	5	90
Workouts 3, 6, 9	4	10	60
C1 Barbell bent-over row			
Workouts 1, 4, 7	2	20	45
Workouts 2, 5, 8	5	5	90
Workouts 3, 6, 9	4	10	60
C2 Barbell incline bench press			
Workouts 1, 4, 7	2	20	45
Workouts 2, 5, 8	5	5	90
Workouts 3, 6, 9	4	10	60
D1 Wood chop	2	15**	45
D2 Three-point plank	2	1*	45

** Each side. Start with your weaker or nondominant side—probably your left if you're right-handed. Don't rest until after you've done all the reps with each side.

* Hold for 45 seconds. Switch legs for the second set.

WORKOUT B (TOTAL BODY)			
Exercise	Sets	Reps	Rest (seconds)
A Jump squat			
Workouts 1, 2, 3	3	5	75
Workouts 4, 5, 6	4	4	75
Workouts 7, 8, 9	5	3	75
B1 Wide-grip pull-up or lat pulldown			
Workouts 1, 4, 7	2	20	45
Workouts 2, 5, 8	5	5	90
Workouts 3, 6, 9	4	10	60
B2 Dumbbell single-arm push press			
Workouts 1, 4, 7	2	20**	45
Workouts 2, 5, 8	5	5	90
Workouts 3, 6, 9	4	10	60
C1 Dumbbell Romanian deadlift			
Workouts 1, 4, 7	2	20	45
Workouts 2, 5, 8	5	5	90
Workouts 3, 6, 9	4	10	60
C2 Bulgarian split squat			
Workouts 1, 4, 7	2	20**	45
Workouts 2, 5, 8	5	5	90
Workouts 3, 6, 9	4	10	60
D1 Reverse crunch	2	20	45
D2 Side plank	2	1*	45

** Each side. Start with your weaker or non-dominant side—probably your left if you're right-handed. Don't rest until after you've done all the reps with each side.

* Hold for 45 seconds on each side. Don't rest until after you've worked both sides.

Phase 2

WORKOUT A (TOTAL BODY)			
Exercise	**Sets**	**Reps**	**Rest (seconds)**
A Barbell clean pull			
Workouts 1, 2, 3	3	5	75
Workouts 4, 5, 6	4	4	75
Workouts 7, 8, 9	5	3	75
B1 Front squat/push press			
Workouts 1, 4, 7	2	20	45
Workouts 2, 5, 8	5	5	90
Workouts 3, 6, 9	4	10	60
B2 Reverse lunge			
Workouts 1, 4, 7	2	20**	45
Workouts 2, 5, 8	5	5	90
Workouts 3, 6, 9	4	10	60
C1 Wide-grip cable row			
Workouts 1, 4, 7	2	20	45
Workouts 2, 5, 8	5	5	90
Workouts 3, 6, 9	4	10	60
C2 Dumbbell bench press			
Workouts 1, 4, 7	2	20	45
Workouts 2, 5, 8	5	5	90
Workouts 3, 6, 9	4	10	60
D1 Reverse wood chop	2	15**	0^^
D2 Side plank	2	1*	60

** Each side. Start with your weaker or nondominant side.

^^Go directly from the first set of reverse wood chops to the side plank without rest.

* Hold for 60 seconds on each side, without resting in between sides. Then rest for 60 seconds and do the second set of reverse wood chops.

WORKOUT B (TOTAL BODY)			
Exercise	Sets	Reps	Rest (seconds)
A Jump lunge			
Workouts 1, 2, 3	3	5**	75
Workouts 4, 5, 6	4	4	75
Workouts 7, 8, 9	5	3	75
B1 Chin-up or underhand-grip lat pulldown			
Workouts 1, 4, 7	2	20	45
Workouts 2, 5, 8	5	5	90
Workouts 3, 6, 9	4	10	60
B2 Barbell push press			
Workouts 1, 4, 7	2	20**	45
Workouts 2, 5, 8	5	5	90
Workouts 3, 6, 9	4	10	60
C1 Supine hip extension/leg curl			
Workouts 1, 4, 7	2	20	45
Workouts 2, 5, 8	5	5	90
Workouts 3, 6, 9	4	10	60
C2 Bulgarian split squat with elevated front foot			
Workouts 1, 4, 7	2	20**	45
Workouts 2, 5, 8	5	5	90
Workouts 3, 6, 9	4	10	60
D1 Swiss-ball crunch	2	20	0^^
D2 Three-point plank	2	1*	60

**Each side. Start with your weaker or nondominant side—probably your left if you're right-handed. Don't rest until after you've done all the reps with each side.

^^Go directly from the first set of Swiss-ball crunches to the plank without rest.

* Hold for 60 seconds. Switch legs for the second set.

SUMMER

If you've been following the *BFS* programs from the beginning, you're bigger, stronger, leaner, and more athletic than you were before you started. Now it's time to put the finishing touches on your physique. You'll continue doing total-body workouts, but you'll add sprints and interval cardio in Phase 1, digging deeper into whatever fat is still holding on and bringing out the topographic contours of your midsection.

You'll also—finally!—get to do some biceps curls and triceps extensions to add a little more display potential to your arm muscles.

These workouts move away from heavy weights with low reps. In Phase 1, you'll do as many as twenty-five reps per set in some of your workouts. It's not because you don't need any more strength or muscle mass—we can all use a little more. And it's not because you're trying to "tone" or "shape" your muscles. The goal here is to confuse the crap out of your body by giving it a different type of stimulus—or, more accurately, to confuse the fat off your body. The shock of new, deeply exhausting work will speed up your metabolism, trimming fat while maintaining your muscle size, and perhaps even adding a bit more of it.

Phase 2 moves on from sprints and intervals into something even more diabolical: giant sets. You'll do four consecutive exercises without resting in between any of them. Then you'll take a short rest and repeat the giant set however many times the workout requires.

There's no sugar-coating this: these Summer workouts are the toughest in the programs. You can't do them right if you aren't willing to focus and work your ass off. But when you finish the program with a body that turns heads on the beach or in your favorite bar, you'll understand why I put you through it, and you'll be happy you pushed yourself to get the results you've always wanted.

Phase 1

WORKOUT A (TOTAL BODY)			
Exercise	**Sets**	**Reps**	**Rest (seconds)**
A1 Squat			
Workouts 1, 4, 7	4	8	60
Workouts 2, 5, 8	2	25	45
Workouts 3, 6, 9	3	15	30
A2 Barbell bent-over row			
Workouts 1, 4, 7	4	8	60
Workouts 2, 5, 8	2	25	45
Workouts 3, 6, 9	3	15	30
A3 Side plank			
Workouts 1, 4, 7	4	1*	60
Workouts 2, 5, 8	2	1†	45
Workouts 3, 6, 9	3	1*	30
B1 Bulgarian split squat			
Workouts 1, 4, 7	4	8‡	60
Workouts 2, 5, 8	2	25	45
Workouts 3, 6, 9	3	15	30
B2 Dumbbell incline bench press or push-up			
Workouts 1, 4, 7	4	8**	60
Workouts 2, 5, 8	2	25	45
Workouts 3, 6, 9	3	15	30
B3 Swiss-ball crunch			
Workouts 1, 4, 7	4	8	60
Workouts 2, 5, 8	2	25	45
Workouts 3, 6, 9	3	15	30

continued on next page

Sprints

You can do these on a stationary bike, or sprint outside if the weather allows it. (Because the intervals are very short, it's impractical to do them on any other type of equipment.)

Warm up for 5 minutes, then go as hard as you can for 10 seconds. Go easy for 20 seconds. That's one round.

Do eight rounds the first week, and add one round per week. By week six, you'll be doing 13 rounds in your final A workout of Phase 1. (Remember, you do the A workout twice in weeks one, three, and five, and once in weeks two, four, and six.)

* Hold for 30 seconds on each side. Don't rest until you've done both sides.

† Hold for 45 seconds on each side. Don't rest until you've done both sides.

‡ Each side. Start with your weaker or nondominant side—probably your left if you're right-handed. Don't rest until after you've done all the reps with each side.

** Do bench presses when the workout specifies 4 x 8. Do push-ups for the higher-repetition sets— the most difficult push-up variation you can do for the number of reps specified.

WORKOUT B (TOTAL BODY)			
Exercise	Sets	Reps	Rest (seconds)
A1 Supine hip extension/leg curl			
Workouts 1, 4, 7	4	8	60
Workouts 2, 5, 8	2	25	45
Workouts 3, 6, 9	3	15	30
A2 Step-up			
Workouts 1, 4, 7	4	8*	60
Workouts 2, 5, 8	2	25	45
Workouts 3, 6, 9	3	15	30
A3 Reverse crunch			
Workouts 1, 4, 7	4	15	60
Workouts 2, 5, 8	2	15	45
Workouts 3, 6, 9	3	15	30

continued on next page

Exercise	Sets	Reps	Rest (seconds)
B1 Wide-grip lat pulldown			
Workouts 1, 4, 7	4	8*	60
Workouts 2, 5, 8	2	25	45
Workouts 3, 6, 9	3	15	30
B2 Barbell push press			
Workouts 1, 4, 7	4	8	60
Workouts 2, 5, 8	2	25	45
Workouts 3, 6, 9	3	15	30
B3 Plank			
Workouts 1, 4, 7	3	1**	60
Workouts 2, 5, 8	2	1**	45
Workouts 3, 6, 9	2	1**	30

Intervals

These intervals are longer than the sprints you did in Workout A, so you can use a treadmill, stationary bike, elliptical machine, or stair-climber indoors, or run or ride a bike outdoors. You can also opt to swim indoors or out, although the timing issue gets tricky—you may find yourself in the middle of a lap when it's time to start or stop an interval.

Warm up for 5 minutes, then go as hard as you can for 1 minute (60 seconds). Go easy for 2 minutes (120 seconds). That's one round.

Do five rounds in all your B workouts the first and second weeks; they should take you 20 minutes, including the warm-up.

Do six rounds the third and fourth weeks, making the interval workouts 23 minutes long.

Do seven rounds the fifth and sixth weeks, which should take you 26 minutes.

* Each side. Start with your weaker or nondominant side—probably your left if you're right-handed. Don't rest until after you've done all the reps with each side.

** When doing three sets of planks (workouts 1, 4, 7), hold 60 seconds in the plank position. When doing two sets, hold 75 seconds.

Phase 2

WORKOUT A (TOTAL BODY)			
Exercise	**Sets**	**Reps**	**Rest (seconds)**
A1 Front squat			
Workouts 1, 4, 7	3	15	0
Workouts 2, 5, 8	4	6	0
Workouts 3, 6, 9	4	12	0
A2 Neutral-grip lat pulldown			
Workouts 1, 4, 7	3	15	0
Workouts 2, 5, 8	4	6	0
Workouts 3, 6, 9	4	12	0
A3 Reverse lunge			
Workouts 1, 4, 7	3	15**	0
Workouts 2, 5, 8	4	6	0
Workouts 3, 6, 9	4	12	0
A4 Dumbbell shoulder press			
Workouts 1, 4, 7	3	15	120
Workouts 2, 5, 8	4	6	120
Workouts 3, 6, 9	4	12	120
B1 Wood chop			
Workouts 1, 4, 7	3	15**	0
Workouts 2, 5, 8	4	6	0
Workouts 3, 6, 9	4	12	0
B2 Barbell reverse curl			
Workouts 1, 4, 7	3	15	0
Workouts 2, 5, 8	4	6	0
Workouts 3, 6, 9	4	12	0
			continued on next page

Exercise	Sets	Reps	Rest (seconds)
B3 Reverse crunch			
Workouts 1, 4, 7	3	15	0
Workouts 2, 5, 8	4	15	0
Workouts 3, 6, 9	4	15	0
B4 Dumbbell alternating curl			
Workouts 1, 4, 7	3	15**	120
Workouts 2, 5, 8	4	6	120
Workouts 3, 6, 9	4	12	120

** Each side. Start with your weaker or nondominant side—probably your left if you're right-handed. Don't rest until after you've done all the reps with each side.

WORKOUT B (TOTAL BODY)			
Exercise	Sets	Reps	Rest (seconds)
A1 Supine hip extension/leg curl			
Workouts 1, 4, 7	3	15	0
Workouts 2, 5, 8	4	6	0
Workouts 3, 6, 9	4	12	0
A2 Swiss-ball crunch			
Workouts 1, 4, 7	3	15	0
Workouts 2, 5, 8	4	6	0
Workouts 3, 6, 9	4	12	0
A3 Wide-grip cable row			
Workouts 1, 4, 7	3	15	0
Workouts 2, 5, 8	4	6	0
Workouts 3, 6, 9	4	12	0

continued on next page

Exercise	Sets	Reps	Rest (seconds)
A4 Dumbbell incline bench press (neutral grip)			
Workouts 1, 4, 7	3	15	120
Workouts 2, 5, 8	4	6	120
Workouts 3, 6, 9	4	12	120
B1 Dumbbell lying triceps extension			
Workouts 1, 4, 7	3	15	0
Workouts 2, 5, 8	4	6	0
Workouts 3, 6, 9	4	12	0
B2 Goblet squat			
Workouts 1, 4, 7	3	15	0
Workouts 2, 5, 8	4	6	0
Workouts 3, 6, 9	4	12	0
B3 Dip			
Workouts 1, 4, 7	3	15	0
Workouts 2, 5, 8	4	15	0
Workouts 3, 6, 9	4	15	0
B4 Reverse wood chop			
Workouts 1, 4, 7	3	15**	120
Workouts 2, 5, 8	4	6	120
Workouts 3, 6, 9	4	12	120

** Each side. Start with your weaker or nondominant side—probably your left if you're right-handed. Don't rest until after you've done all the reps with each side.

CHAPTER EIGHT

The *Built for Show* Exercises

WIDE-GRIP CABLE ROW

The goods

Rowing exercises hit all your major upper-back muscles—latissimus dorsi, trapezius, the rear part of your deltoids—as well as your biceps and forearms. But I like to think of rows in terms of their potential for building your traps.

Your trapezius is a four-cornered sheet of thick, strong muscle that links the backs of your shoulders with the base of your skull and the middle of your spine. It has three basic actions: it can pull your shoulder blades together, as it does in this exercise; lift them, as it does in a shrug; or pull them down, as in a chin-up or lat pulldown.

I focus on your traps with many of the key exercises in *BFS* for a simple reason: When the trapezius is fully developed, there is no muscle on your body that makes your shoulders look wider, your back look thicker, and your neck look less like something you'd use to fill in those little circles on standardized tests.

The gear

You'll need a cable apparatus, which is no problem if you work out in a commercial gym, which will have at least one station dedicated to seated cable rows. I want you to use a long bar, which you'll probably have to take from the lat-pulldown station. If you can't get that bar, just use the bar that allows you to take the widest possible overhand grip.

How to do it

Sit on the bench with your knees bent and feet on the supports. Grab the bar overhand with a grip that's substantially greater than shoulder width. I don't want to get super-specific here, since arm length varies so much from one lifter to the next, so I'll just say that the grip should be wide enough for you to notice that it's *unusually* wide. Sit up straight so you're holding the bar with your arms straight and some tension in the cable.

Now pull the bar to your midsection, feeling a good squeeze in your shoulder blades at the end. Return to the starting position and repeat.

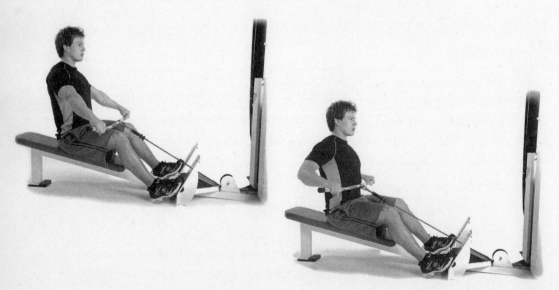

THE GARAGE VARIATION: No cable machine? No problem. Just do a barbell bent-over row (see page 126).

DON'T BE THAT GUY: You want to keep your torso upright throughout the exercise—don't rock back and forth like you're pulling an oar on a slave ship. And please don't be the guy who lets the weight plates on the cable stack slam down into each other at the end of the set. You don't need attention that badly, do you?

NOTE: We shot the *BFS* exercises at a really, really cool athlete-training facility called Velocity Sports in Allentown, Pennsylvania. They turned us loose and let us use everything in any way we needed it. But because it's a serious sports-training facility, some of the equipment doesn't look like what you'd find in a typical health club. So if you notice that the seated-row station in our photos looks different from the one in your gym, that's why. Just use what you have with the form I describe.

DUMBBELL BENCH PRESS

The goods

Everyone knows that a bench press hits your pectoral muscles, and we all love our pecs. Just as important, though, is the fact that chest presses also develop the front part of your deltoid muscles and your triceps. If you work hard on chest presses (along with shoulder presses, described later in this chapter), you shouldn't need a lot of extra work for your shoulders and arms; they'll develop just fine as you get stronger and use heavier weights.

The gear

Just dumbbells and a bench—couldn't be much simpler.

How to do it

To get in position, sit on a bench and place the dumbbells on your thighs. Using your legs to help, push the weights up to your shoulders as you lower yourself back onto the bench. In the starting position, you want the back of your head, your shoulder blades, and your butt touching the bench. Your lower back is slightly arched—it shouldn't be flat on the bench. Your feet should be at least shoulder-width apart and flat on the floor. Hold the dumbbells with an over-hand grip with your thumbs facing each other and the weights touching your outer chest.

Push the weights straight up until your arms are fully extended. The weights shouldn't touch when they're over your chest, or really come close to touching. Lower them to your chest, and repeat.

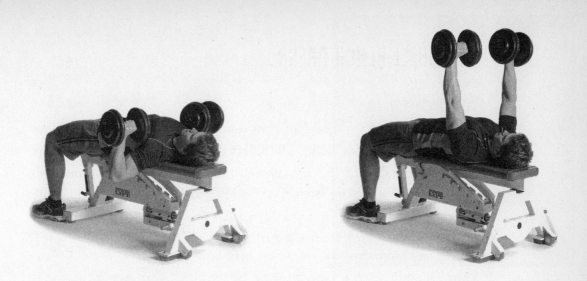

THE GARAGE VARIATION: Few homeschooled lifters have the luxury of a full set of fixed-weight dumbbells, like you'll find in a gym. You can buy good selectorized dumbbell sets—the kind that let you adjust the weight of a single set of dumbbells up or down as easily as you select weights on a cable machine. (Power-Block is the best-known brand; others include Bowflex, Ironmaster, and Versa-Bell.) But those cost a couple hundred bucks per pair and typically max out at fifty pounds; to go heavier, it'll cost more.

Conventional adjustable dumbbells—handles, weight plates, collars to hold the weights in place—are a lot cheaper, but also time-consuming and clunky to use.

So at this point you probably expect me to say, "Yeah, go ahead and use a barbell." But I have a better idea: If you can't get two dumbbells, use one. That's right—do bench presses exactly as I describe them above, but using one arm at a time. (Put your nonworking hand on your midsection.) Start with your non-dominant arm (your left if you're right-handed), and then do the same number of reps with your dominant side.

DON'T BE THAT GUY: Why not a barbell bench press? Because guys put way too much emphasis on it, particularly on how much weight they use. For a lot of lifters, there's a safety issue—it's hard on the shoulders (usually the right shoulder, if you're right-handed). But even if there isn't, there's a "bro" issue. As in, all the bro-tards gather around the barbell bench-press station in the gym, shouting "all you!" to a buddy as they pull the bar off his chest when they realize he can't actually lift it. (Obviously, it's not "all you" unless you're lifting the bar with no help from your spotters. They shouldn't touch the bar if you're going to claim the lift as a personal record.)

Really, it doesn't matter how much you can bench press, especially if your attempt at a bigger max ruins your shoulders or annoys everyone else in the gym. Dumbbells force your arms to work independently, which is easier on your shoulders and promotes better muscular balance.

Note: If I don't specify a specific angle for the bench, that means it should be flat—the default setting.

CHIN-UP

The goods

If you want the biggest biceps your genetics allow, master this exercise. As I said in Chapter 2, there's no difference between what your biceps do in a chin-up and what they do in a curl. Except of course, for the amount of work they do. Pulling your body's full weight repeatedly through a range of motion presents your biceps with a lot more work than you'd ever give them on a curl. Granted, most of the work is being done by your lats, the bigger and stronger mid-back muscles, especially at the beginning of the exercise. But you can't pull yourself up to that bar without your biceps pitching in (try it with straight arms if you don't believe me), and that means your biceps are taking on a much bigger load than you'd ever give them if you were curling a barbell or dumbbells.

Conveniently, chin-ups are also great for your lats, which give your torso that nice V-shaped taper that all of us want.

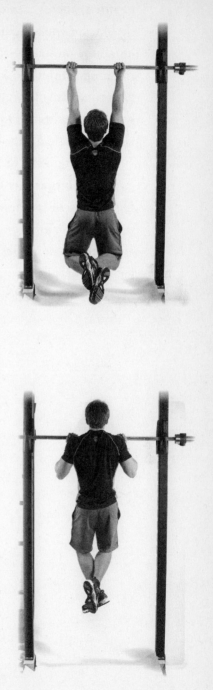

The gear

Just a chin-up bar and your body.

How to do it

Grab the bar underhand with your hands slightly less than shoulder-width apart. Start each rep at a dead hang, and then pull yourself up until your chin passes the bar.

THE GARAGE VARIATION: Your best choice is a fixed bar. If you get a power cage for squats, the top crossbar works perfectly as a chin-up bar. Be careful with those twist-in or screw-in bars you put in or over doorways. It needs to be sturdy, allowing you to work hard without fear that the bar will rip out of the doorway halfway through a repetition. Plus, the twist-in bars can mess up a doorway; you should get permission from your wife, landlord, roommates, or parents before you take that risk.

DON'T BE THAT GUY: A lot of muscles come into play when you're trying to keep your body steady while you pull it up and lower it. Muscles in your lower back, glutes, and thighs are important stabilizers. But some guys get their abs and hip flexors into the act, raising their knees to generate momentum on each rep. These guys also tend to "short-arm" their reps, starting each chin-up with their arms already half-bent, instead of going from a dead hang.

Note: If you can't do chin-ups for the number of reps specified in the workout charts, do underhand-grip lat pulldowns instead. If you work out at a gym, you can also use the assisted chin-up machine, although I confess I'm not a big fan.

UNDERHAND-GRIP LAT PULLDOWN

The goods

Pulldowns work the same muscles as chin-ups. The big difference is that they're easier, and less challenging to your muscles. So this is a perfectly fine fall-back exercise when you can't do chin-ups for the designated number of reps, but chin-ups are always the first choice, especially on low-rep sets.

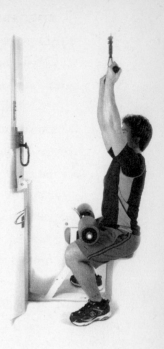

The gear

A cable apparatus with a high pulley and a straight bar that allows you to use an underhand grip.

How to do it

Grab the bar with an underhand grip that's just inside shoulder width. Set your knees underneath the support pad. (The less you rely on the pad, the more you use your core muscles for balance and stability, and the more you get out of the exercise.) Starting with straight arms, pull the bar down to the top of your chest, briefly making contact with your chest and squeezing your shoulder blades together. Return to the starting position and repeat.

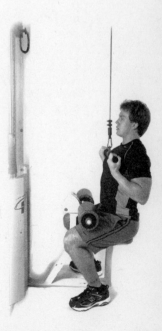

THE GARAGE VARIATION: There's no perfect substitution for lat pulldowns. But reverse push-ups, aka horizontal chin-ups, come pretty close. Set up a barbell across two sturdy supports so it's about three feet off the floor. Get under the bar and grab it underhand, with your hands just inside shoulder width. Straighten your body so your heels touch the floor and your body forms a straight line from neck to ankles, as it would for a push-up. From there, pull yourself up as high as you can, lower yourself, and repeat. Pay close attention to your posture; you want to keep your back in its natural alignment throughout.

If you can't rig a setup like that, you can do underhand-grip bent-over rows with a barbell or dumbbells (see page 126).

DON'T BE THAT GUY: It's okay to lean back slightly on this exercise, but only if you keep that position throughout the range of motion. If you need to lean back in the middle of a rep, what you're really doing is pulling the bar with an action called "hip extension"—you're using lower-body muscles to help you do an upper-body exercise.

Note: A better technique is to push your chest out toward the bar, which forces your shoulders back and gives your upper-back muscles a greater range of motion to work with.

DUMBBELL SHOULDER PRESS WITH NEUTRAL GRIP

The goods

Everyone knows the shoulder press is a "shoulder" exercise—kind of hard to miss that nuance when it's right there in the name. And it certainly hits the front and middle parts of the deltoid muscles. But, like the dumbbell bench press, it's also a highly underrated exercise for your triceps. Your delts are the prime movers, since it's their job to pull your upper arms up overhead. But triceps, and only triceps, straighten your elbows when they're bent, and without straightened arms there's no shoulder press. Your upper traps also contribute, since they're involved in lifting your shoulder blades.

The gear

Just dumbbells.

How to do it

Hold the dumbbells just above your deltoids with a neutral grip (palms facing each other). Your elbows will be in front of your torso, pointing forward (more or less). Press the dumbbells straight up from your shoulders. Keep your torso in the same basic alignment; don't arch backward or look up at the weights as you lift them. Return to the starting position and repeat.

THE GARAGE VARIATION: As with the bench press, if you can't put together two dumbbells, do it with one arm at a time.

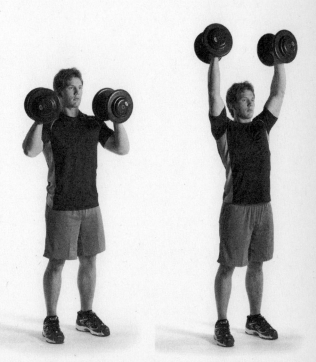

DON'T BE THAT GUY: Gym culture, for some reason, seems to have accepted the bodybuilding-world notion that the only way to do a shoulder press is seated, with your upper back braced against a vertical support. I'm not sure if the idea is that this is safer, or if it's seen as being a stricter challenge to your shoulder muscles. Either way, it's bogus. Stand up and use your own body for balance and support. Work hard enough and your muscles will be completely challenged.

Note: Why a neutral grip, instead of the traditional position, in which your hands are on the same line, as if you were using a barbell? It's easier on the shoulders for most guys, since your upper arms start out in front of your torso, rather than even with or slightly behind it. That opens the shoulder capsule a bit, reducing the potential for friction and impingement. Not that there's anything inherently dangerous about the traditional shoulder-press grip—you'll use it later in the program.

REVERSE CRUNCH

The goods
Abs, anyone?

The gear
If you have a floor, you're good to go.

How to do it
Lie on your back on the floor. Lift your legs off the floor with your hips and knees bent 90 degrees—that is, your thighs are perpendicular to the floor and your lower legs are parallel to it. Set your hands on the floor, palms down.

Contract your abs and curl your hips up off the floor. Imagine you have a pitcher of water on your knees, and you're trying to pour the water onto your chest. "Unroll" your spine to reverse the movement and return to the starting position. Try to avoid using momentum here; start each rep from a complete stop.

THE GARAGE VARIATION: You might want to put something over that oil stain on the floor before you lie down on it.

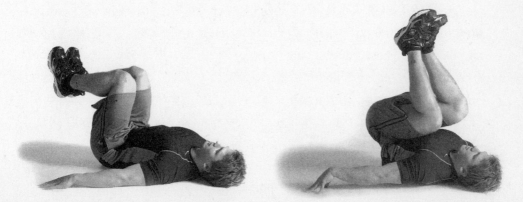

PLANK

The goods

The plank is so clearly a yoga-based move that most guys, in my experience, have trouble accepting that it's one of the best exercises on earth for your abdominals. That is, until they actually try it. I've seen some very, very strong and fit guys shake like they're having an epileptic fit in the middle of an earthquake before they hit the one-minute mark on their first-ever plank.

Most of us who aspire to be built for show think of ab training as something you do that's active—a crunch or sit-up, a side crunch, a hanging leg raise (the advanced version of the reverse crunch). No argument from me; those exercises absolutely work the abdominal muscles, especially the rectus abdominis, the six-pack muscle. But most of the work your abs do in real life involves a *lack* of movement.

Let me back up a bit: your abdominal wall actually has four layers of muscle. The innermost layer, the transverse abdominis, protects your internal organs. The next layer, your internal obliques, helps with all the movements of your trunk (twisting, bending, crunching). Its most important job, though, is postural. It keeps you upright. Your external obliques do the heavy-duty twisting and crunching, and your rectus abdominis does the obvious crunching while protecting everything else during twists.

Of all those movements, the one that you do most often is sit or stand up straight. Even when you're lifting weights, you still have to maintain your postural integrity. You have to be able to brace your midsection to do front squats and deadlifts. Those muscles come into play in virtually every exercise in *Built for Show*, from seated cable rows to standing shoulder presses. You're using your mid-body muscles on chin-ups to keep your body steady as you hang from the bar, and you can't do a good bench press without tightening your belly to provide a strong platform.

That's why the plank, which involves holding a single position for a designated period of time, is such an important exercise: it teaches your midsection muscles to work hard and maintain your body's alignment even when you aren't moving.

The gear
The floor's the limit.

How to do it
Lie facedown on the floor, with your weight resting on your forearms and toes. Your elbows are directly below your shoulders, and your feet are shoulder-width apart. Your body should be straight from neck to ankles. Tighten up your abs and hold for the time designated.

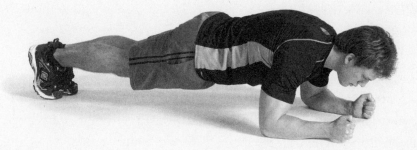

THE GARAGE VARIATION: Make sure that you have really good padding beneath your elbows. You'll destroy them if you try to do this on a bare concrete floor.

FRONT SQUAT

The goods

Most gym veterans consider the traditional back squat the king of all exercises—it allows you to use heavier weights than just about any exercise (although some guys, particularly if they have relatively long arms, can deadlift more than they can squat). It also works more muscles, and works them harder.

But most of the strength coaches I know prefer the front squat over the back squat, despite the fact that all of us can lift more weight if it's across the back of our shoulders, rather than resting on the front. That's because the front squat forces you to lift with a more upright torso, and allows a great range of motion for the hips and knees. It also puts less compressive force on your spine, and tends to be easier on your back and knees.

The benefits are huge: you work all your lower-body muscles as hard as they can be worked, although you'll probably feel it most directly in your quadriceps, the muscles on the front of your thighs. Your mid-body muscles also get a serious challenge—your abs and lower back have crucial stabilizing duties, while your hip muscles work through a full range of motion.

The gear

You need a barbell and a squat rack or power cage—something sturdy that allows you to start with the bar at about shoulder level.

How to do it

Set the bar in a power cage so it's at about chest level. Grab the bar in an overhand grip with your hands just slightly beyond shoulder width. Lift your elbows so your upper arms are parallel to the floor and the bar rests on the front of your shoulders, making very gentle contact with your neck. To hold this position, you'll probably need to roll the bar off your palms so you're holding it with your fingers.

Now lift the bar off the supports and step back so your feet are shoulder-width apart and your toes are pointed forward or angled out slightly. Push your hips back and descend into a squat, keeping your torso upright and your feet flat on the floor. Go as deep as possible, then push back up to the starting position and repeat.

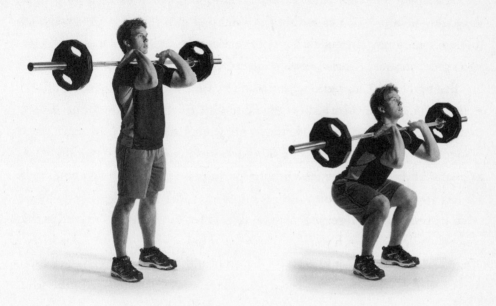

THE GARAGE VARIATION: This is why you need a squat rack or power cage in your home gym. Without one, you'll have to start the exercise with the bar on the floor, as described on page 116.

DON'T BE THAT GUY: With the back squat, a lot of guys get into the habit of descending halfway on each rep. It allows them to lift heavier weights, and then claim bragging rights. The front squat takes away the temptation to cheat. You can't use as much weight, and even if you could nobody cares how much you can lift on a front squat. So do yourself a favor and use a full range of motion, with the tops of your thighs slightly below parallel to the floor in the bottom position.

Note: To make it easier to see my form on the exercise, I didn't want to clutter up the photos with a lot of extraneous gear. But if I were just doing this exercise in my regular workout, of course I'd use a power cage. The cage serves two purposes:

First, you get to start with the weight already up at shoulder level. Otherwise, you'd have to pick it up off the floor and pull it to your shoulders—a move that's so technically complex it's actually an exercise by itself: the power clean. It's called a "power" clean to distinguish it from the regular clean, which is the first half of the clean and jerk, which is an Olympic weight-lifting move. (To do a clean, you pick up a barbell off the floor and "catch" it on the front of your shoulders as you lower your body into a full front squat.)

Second, you can set the cage's side supports a couple feet above the floor. That way, if you get stuck in the bottom position on a repetition, you can leave the bar on the safety supports and get out from under it with your body intact (even if your pride suffers a momentary setback).

STEP-UP

The goods

If you're doing these right, you'll build all your lower-body muscles while also making sure you develop balanced strength in both legs.

The gear

You need a barbell and a sturdy step that's at least twelve inches high. The higher the step, the harder each rep will be.

How to do it

Set the barbell on supports in a power cage so it's at about shoulder height. (If you've done back squats, use that same setting for the supports.) Approach it backward, and grab the bar with an overhand grip with your hands just wider than shoulder width. Squeeze your shoulder blades together, and rest the bar on the little shelf you create with your upper-back muscles. Lift the bar off the rack and walk up to your step.

Place one foot on the step (start with your right if you're left-handed), with the foot flat. Push down with that foot and raise your body until you're standing straight and your trailing foot touches the step. Immediately lower your trailing foot back to the floor and start the next rep. After you finish your reps, switch legs and repeat.

At no point should you push off from the floor with your nonworking leg; it's just along for the ride here.

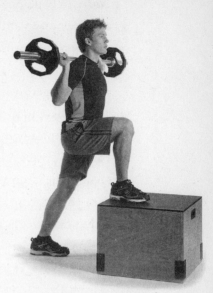

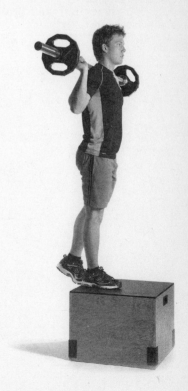

THE GARAGE VARIATION: You probably won't have a lot to choose from in terms of steps. Just make sure that whatever you use—milk crate, bench, toolbox—is sturdy enough to held your weight, and has a surface that your feet won't slide off of.

DON'T BE THAT GUY: Think this is a girly exercise? Try using a higher step and a heavier weight. Yeah, you feel it now, don't you?

Note: You can also do this exercise holding dumbbells at your sides. It's a little easier, but easier isn't better. Having the weight on your shoulders makes it more of a total-body challenge. And when you're holding dumbbells, your grip might give out while your legs still have a few reps left in them.

SUPINE HIP EXTENSION/LEG CURL

The goods

This exercise is to your gluteals what the bench press is to your pecs. You can't really target your buttock muscles much more directly than you do here. As a bonus, you also work your hamstrings and strengthen your lower back. You also work your calves, since they get called into action to assist your hamstrings on the "leg curl" part of the exercise, because your hamstrings are already assisting your glutes on the "hip extension."

The gear

A floor and a Swiss ball.

How to do it

Since there's something of a learning curve on this exercise, I've broken it down into three levels of difficulty. Many of you will be able to start with Level 2, but it's not a problem if you have to begin with Level 1. Just move up as soon as you can. Many of you will never get to Level 3, but that's okay too. As long as you remain challenged with Level 2, you'll get all the intended benefits.

LEVEL 1: Lie on your back with your feet flat on top of a Swiss ball, knees bent. Your hips are on the floor. Spread your arms out away from your torso, palms down, for balance. Push down through your heels and lift your hips off the floor until your body forms a straight line from knees to shoulders. Feel the squeeze in your glutes, then lower your hips until they come close to the floor but don't actually touch it. Do the rest of your reps, and don't let your butt touch the floor until after the last rep of the set.

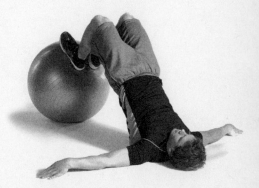

LEVEL 2: When that's easy, it's time to add in the leg curl. The setup is the same, except that your legs are straight and only your heels are on the ball. Start with the hip extension, pushing down through your heels and lifting your hips off the floor until your body forms a straight line from your ankles to your shoulders.

Now pull the ball toward your body with your feet until your feet are flat on the ball, your knees are bent about 90 degrees, and your body forms a straight line from your knees to your shoulders.

Pause, feel the squeeze in your glutes and hamstrings, and lower your hips toward the floor as you roll the ball back to the starting position. As in Level 1, don't let your hips rest on the floor between reps.

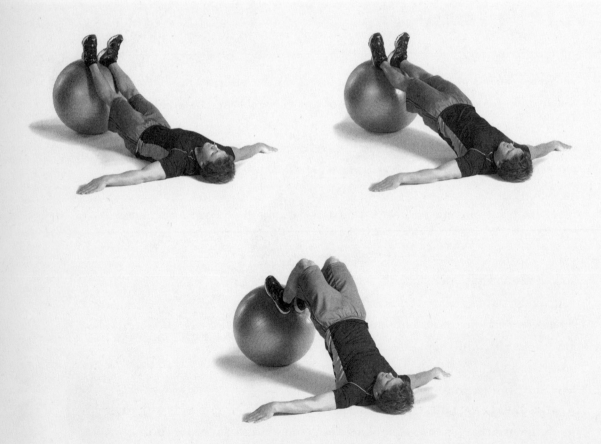

LEVEL 3: Start as you would for Level 2, with the hip extension. Lift one foot off the ball and bend that knee 90 degrees. Now curl the ball using your other leg. Roll the ball back to the starting position, but keep your hips up and your nonworking leg up in the air. Do all your reps as leg curls from that position, then switch legs and repeat the set.

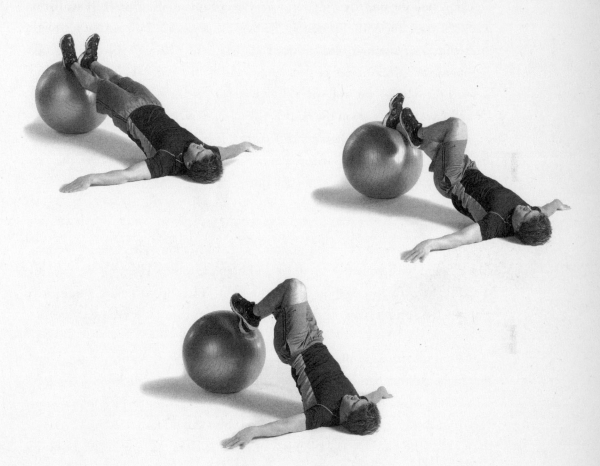

THE GARAGE VARIATION: No Swiss ball? You can do the hip extension with your heels up on a chair. If you get a rolling chair, you can also do the leg curl.

CABLE WOOD CHOP

The goods

Your abs—particularly your obliques on the sides of your waist—are responsible for bending and twisting, and here you'll do some of both. If you play baseball, tennis, or golf, this exercise helps increase your rotational power, turning singles into doubles, doubles into homers, and 250-yard drives into 300-yard bombs.

The gear

You'll need a cable apparatus with a rope attachment. In most gyms, you'd do this on the cable-crossover machine, although you can also use the lat-pulldown station. Any high cable will do.

How to do it

Stand sideways to the cable station, with your right side close to the machine. Stand with your feet shoulder-width apart, toes pointed forward, knees flexed slightly. Turn your shoulders to the right, reach up with both hands, and grab the rope attachment. Turn your head with your shoulders so your eyes are on the rope.

Now pull the rope diagonally down and across your torso, rotating your shoulders as your hands end up on the outside of your left knee. Your eyes should follow the rope through the entire range of motion, which allows your head to turn along with your shoulders. Your hips should face the same direction throughout the movement, keeping your lower back in a strong, stable position while your shoulders rotate. It's okay to pivot on the ball of your right foot, if that's a natural movement pattern for you.

Return to the starting position, finish your reps, then reverse your position and repeat the set.

THE GARAGE VARIATION: For a thoroughly mediocre variation, you can lie on your back with your feet off the floor and pull a ball diagonally across your torso, starting above your right shoulder and ending at your left knee.

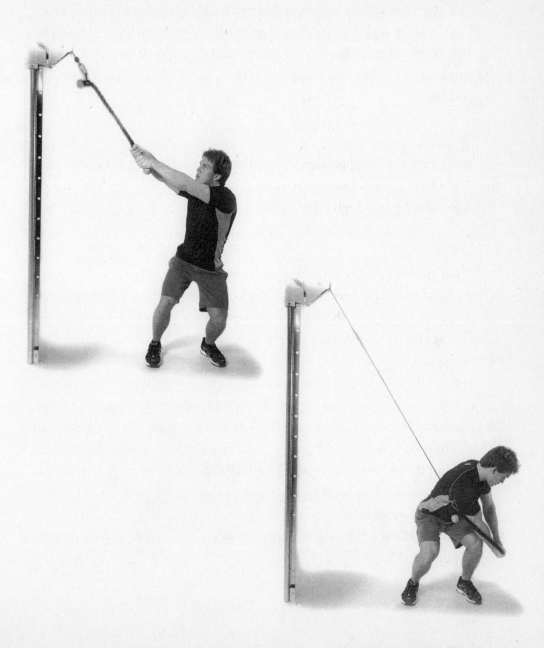

SIDE PLANK

The goods

Another great move for core strength, stability, and endurance. I like to joke that side planks turn love handles into "mah handles"—muscles that make a convenient point of contact during your bedroom workouts. But, as you probably know if you actually have love handles, no single ab exercise burns enough fat to make them disappear. (That's why you need the entire *Built for Show* program to get the results you want.)

Side planks do something more interesting: they improve the performance of the muscles in your midsection, including your obliques and the smaller muscles that provide support to your pelvis and lower back. Should you find yourself in an intimate situation with someone who's the adventurous type, you'll appreciate the strength and stamina you develop with this exercise and the other midsection moves I've included. As the saying goes, you get only one chance to make a good first impression, and it goes double for your first time in bed with a new partner.

The gear

More on the floor.

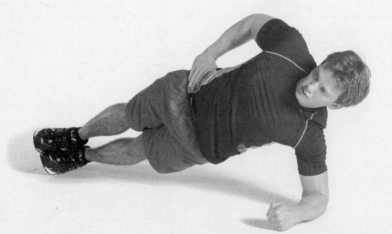

How to do it

Lie on your left side, with your weight resting on your left forearm and the outside edge of your left foot. Your elbow should be directly below your shoulder, and your right foot should be against your left foot, with the inside edges touching, and off the floor. Your body should form a straight line from your neck to your ankles. Put your right hand on your right hip. Hold that position for the designated time.

BARBELL BENT-OVER ROW WITH UNDERHAND GRIP

The goods

As with any rowing exercise, you'll work your traps, lats, and rear delts, along with the smaller and deeper muscles that surround and work with those muscles in your shoulders and upper back. You'll also work your biceps directly, thanks to the underhand grip. The bent-over position adds stabilizing work for all the muscles of your torso, hips, and lower body.

So, really, it's a full-body exercise. Some big, strong muscles are responsible for the heavy lifting, and you'll like the way they respond to bent-over rows by getting bigger and stronger. But just about all the other muscles have to work to support your body as it pulls heavy weights.

If you can't visualize how that might help you become a bedroom samurai, you may be the rare American male who hasn't watched enough porn.

The gear

Just a barbell.

How to do it

Stand with your feet shoulder-width apart, toes pointed forward, knees bent slightly. Grab the barbell underhand, with your hands just slightly wider than

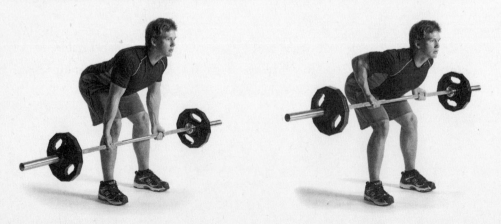

your shoulders. Lift the bar off the floor or supports and hold it with arms fully extended just below the knees. Push your hips back as you fold your torso forward, keeping your midsection tight and your lower back in its natural arch. Your torso won't be parallel to the floor, but the angle of your torso relative to the floor should be 45 degrees or less.

Pull the bar straight up to your upper abdominal area, lower it until your arms are straight, and repeat.

THE GARAGE VARIATION: This is one of those exercises where it helps to have a mirror to check your form. If you don't have one, look around at yard sales (or in your parents' basement, if that's an option).

DON'T BE THAT GUY: I haven't said much (if anything) about using props like a weight belt and lifting straps. But if you work out in a gym that attracts serious bodybuilders, you've probably seen guys using lifting straps for every exercise that involves pulling, especially barbell bent-over rows. Inevitably, those guys are also wearing leather belts.

I want you to avoid using them. Your midsection is the only belt you need; develop strength and stability in those lower-torso muscles and you won't need any additional support. Same with lifting straps. Your hands and wrists should be strong enough to allow you to pull any weight that your back can support.

The goal is to develop *balanced* total-body strength. If some muscles are functionally stronger than others, you've got a problem. Using belts and straps only makes it worse.

Note: At any angle, your back and hips should feel strong and stable. At no point should you feel strain in your lower back. It's okay to lower your hips more and bend your knees more to get that feeling of stability.

DUMBBELL INCLINE BENCH PRESS

The goods

Pectoral muscles have separate upper, middle, and lower portions. According to bodybuilding theology, incline bench presses develop the upper pecs, flat bench presses develop the middle pecs, and decline presses and dips hit the lower portion. (For the record, pecs don't have "inner" and "outer" portions that can be targeted with exercises like close- or wide-grip bench presses.) In reality, those distinctions are meaningless from a functional point of view. All three sections work together, and you can't isolate any one section. The best way to build your chest is with exercises that allow you to use the heaviest possible weights.

So why include incline presses, since you can lift heavier weights on a flat bench? The main reason is to give your shoulders a break by letting them support and move the weights at a different angle. You'll probably give your upper pecs and the front part of your deltoids a slightly bigger challenge than they get in flat bench presses, but I doubt if you'll notice any real difference in your physique when you shift from one to the other.

The gear

You'll need dumbbells and a bench that inclines.

How to do it

Set the bench to a 30-degree angle, relative to the floor. (You can go slightly higher or lower—between 45 and 15 degrees—if you prefer. When in doubt, choose the angle that feels most natural for your shoulder joints.) Grab the dumbbells with an overhand grip and raise them to your shoulders, as described for the dumbbell bench press (page 102), and lie with your back flat against the pad with the weights at the outside edges of your shoulders. Push the weights straight up until your arms are straight and perpendicular to the floor. Lower them to your shoulders and repeat.

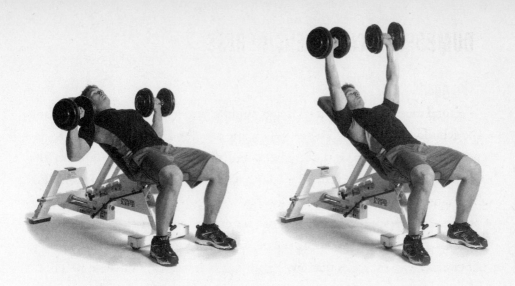

THE GARAGE VARIATION: No incline bench? One easy trick is to put weight plates under one end of the bench, raising it a few inches off the floor. But that, at best, might give you a 15-degree angle; go any higher, and you probably won't have a very stable setup.

Another option, if you can't afford an adjustable bench but you have good carpentry skills and access to cheap lumber, is to make an old-school incline bench. Back before there were such things as adjustable benches, lifters used to rig up planks at a 45-degree angle to the floor. (If you remember the seesaws commonly found in playgrounds before Americans turned litigious, you get an idea of the type of planks they used: eight to twelve inches wide, at least an inch thick, durable and sturdy.) Lifters would back up to the board, and then flop back against it as they hoisted the weights to their shoulders. They could then set their feet on the floor, with their shoulders and butt braced against the board.

It wasn't pretty, but it worked.

WIDE-GRIP LAT PULLDOWN

The goods

As with any variation on the lat pulldown, the focus here is on your lats, while also working your traps, rear delts, biceps, and forearms. The wide grip puts your pulling muscles at a disadvantage, limiting the amount of assistance your lats can receive from your trapezius. So, on the one hand, it's a more direct challenge to your lat muscles. But since the wide grip limits your range of motion and forces you to use slightly less weight, whatever advantage you get from the extra focus on your lats dissipates with the smaller workload.

Mainly, I like to use the wide-grip pulldown because it challenges your muscles and connective tissues in a different way. If you have weak links, using the same grip all the time will probably make the problem worse. Using a variety of grips will help you balance the strength of the muscles and connective tissues in your back and shoulders before any weakness or imbalance becomes a problem for you.

The gear

Every gym has a lat-pulldown station, and most of the time you'll find the long bar already in place.

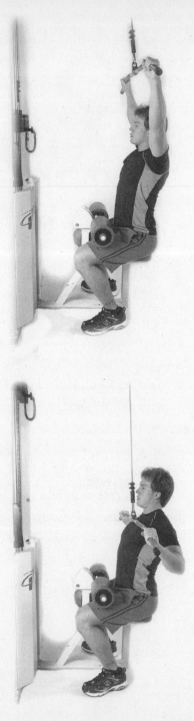

How to do it

Grab the bar with an overhand grip, your hands as wide as you can comfortably manage. The rest of the setup is the same as for the underhand-grip lat pulldown (see page 107). Pull the bar down to the top of your chest as you squeeze your shoulder blades together.

THE GARAGE VARIATION: As I said earlier, there's no perfect substitute for lat pulldowns if you don't have a cable machine. You can try barbell bent-over rows using a wide grip, or the reverse push-ups I described on page 107.

DIP

The goods

In the bodybuilding world, the dip builds your lower pecs along with your triceps and front deltoids. But in the real world, it does a lot more than that. Try this experiment: place your right hand over your left pec. Lift your left arm up and back, with your elbow bent. Now push down with your left arm, imitating the range of motion of a dip. Feel your chest muscles with your right hand. As you can tell, there's a lot more than the lower pecs working. And that's without any resistance. Imagine how hard your pecs will work when they're pushing your entire body weight. For that matter, think of how much harder your triceps work on this exercise than they would if you were doing triceps pushdowns on a cable machine, using maybe a quarter of your body weight. This is one kick-ass upper-body muscle builder.

The gear

You'll need dip bars, which are harder than ever to find in commercial gyms. Even in Velocity, where we shot these photos, we didn't know they had dip bars until a trainer told us where to find them and how to attach them to the power cage. (Thanks, Chris!)

A lot of gyms now have an assistance machine for chin-ups and dips—if you can't use your own body weight, you kneel on a platform and only use as much of your weight as you handle. The platform also folds down, which allows you to use the machine's bars for unassisted chins and dips. (In my experience, the machines tend to be pretty good for unassisted dips, but not so good for traditional chin-ups and pull-ups.)

How to do it

Grab the parallel bars with your knuckles to the outside (an overhand grip). If the bars are adjustable, you probably want to choose the narrower hand position, which should leave your hands just wider than your shoulders. (The wider you go, the tougher it will be for your shoulder joints.) Lift yourself off the floor so your arms are straight, with all your weight resting on your hands. Your body leans forward slightly, your knees are bent, and your lower legs are crossed at the ankles.

Lower yourself until your upper arms are parallel to the floor, then push yourself back up to the starting position and repeat.

If you can easily get the designated number of reps with your body weight, you need to add an external load. Since it's not very practical to put rocks in your pockets, the best choice is a chin-dip belt. This looks like a regular weight belt, but it has a chain in front that allows you to add a dumbbell or weight plates. When you're doing dips with the belt, the weight will dangle in front of you directly below your shoulders.

A slightly more awkward version is to hold a dumbbell between your feet.

THE GARAGE VARIATION: If you have a power cage, I highly recommend getting dip bars that attach to the cage. I've also seen dip bars that attach to heavy-duty barbell bench-press stations. If those aren't realistic options, the next-best choice is a freestanding chin-up/dip station, which you can find at any online store specializing in strength-training equipment.

Lots of guys who work out at home choose "none of the above," and resort to using an exercise called bench dips: sit on the edge of a flat bench, palms on the bench at the sides of your buttocks, fingers curled around the edge of the bench for support. Your legs

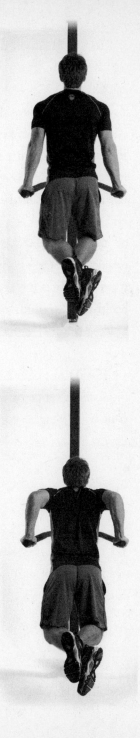

are straight, heels on the floor. (You can also rest your heels on a box or chair so they're off the floor, making it slightly harder.) To do the exercise, lift your butt off the bench, lower it until your upper arms are parallel to the floor, then push back up.

The downside is that it's tough on your shoulders to move your body weight in that position. If you try it and it feels like it's taking a toll on your shoulder joints, try something else, like push-ups with your hands on two boxes. That allows you to work your chest through a longer range of motion than you'd achieve with regular push-ups, with less strain on your most vulnerable joints.

DON'T BE THAT GUY: It takes a while to get the hang of dips, if you've never done them before. Some of you won't be strong enough to use the full range of motion at first. It's okay to do them with a shortened range of motion while you build your strength and improve your technique. It's also okay to use the assistance machine if you can't get all the designated reps using your full body weight.

But it's not okay to dangle a bunch of extra weights from a dip belt while using a short range of motion. If you can't master the full range of motion with your body weight, you aren't ready to add that external load.

DEADLIFT

The goods

I suggested earlier in this chapter that the supine hip extension/leg curl is to the buttocks what the bench press is to the chest. I didn't mean to slight the deadlift, which targets the same muscles with much, much bigger weights. The deadlift hits as much as 75 percent of your body's muscle mass, with the hardest work occurring in what exercise scientists call the posterior chain: hamstrings, glutes, lower back, traps. If you're one of those guys who looks okay from the front and back but disappears when viewed from the side, this exercise is guaranteed to thicken your body from any angle.

The gear

Barbell, floor. You might also want to get some chalk to help you grip the bar without resorting to lifting straps. You can find it for a couple bucks at just about any store that specializes in strength-training equipment.

How to do it

Stand with your shins touching the bar and your feet shoulder-width apart. Push your hips back, reach down, and grab the bar overhand, your arms just outside your legs. Set yourself so your arms are straight, the bar is directly below your shoulders, your hips are back, your lower back is flat (your spine retains its natural arch, but it looks flat), and your knees are bent as much as they need to be. You should feel slight tension in your hamstrings as you get ready to lift. Now tighten up the middle of your body; you should feel as if your pelvis, lower back, and ribs are locked together.

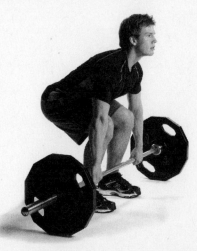

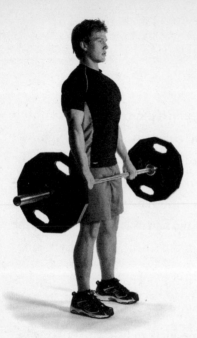

Push down through the middle of the feet and pull the bar straight up your legs. Finish the movement by driving your hips forward and shoulders back.

Control the weight on the way down to the floor; you don't want it to slam on the floor, but at the same time you don't want to waste your energy by making the descent any slower than it needs to be. Let the weight come to a complete rest on the floor before you start the next repetition. With really heavy weights and low reps, you probably want to reset your grip on each rep while the weight is on the floor.

THE GARAGE VARIATION: A deadlift is a deadlift no matter where you do it. The advantage of lifting at home is that you can make more noise.

DON'T BE THAT GUY: Conversely, if you're in a crowded gym, you should be considerate and avoid making excessive exertion-related noise.

BULGARIAN SPLIT SQUAT

The goods

This is hands down the most hated exercise in my studio. It's awkward, it's uncomfortable, it's exhausting, and it doesn't even allow you the satisfaction of using heavy weights. So why do I use it in my workouts? Because it's effective. It builds lower-body muscle, it burns calories, and it does wonders for your overall conditioning. You'll be shocked at how much it improves your overall stamina and ability to work hard. After a few weeks of Bulgarian split squats, everything else feels easier than it used to.

The gear

Dumbbells, a bench or step to rest one foot, and a pair of balls to help you get through it.

How to do it

Grab a pair of dumbbells with an overhand grip and stand about three feet in front of a bench with your back to it, holding the dumbbells at your sides. Place your right foot on the bench behind you, with the top of your foot on the bench. (Some prefer to do it with the ball of their foot on the bench, but I think it makes the exercise more awkward than it needs to be.) Your left foot is flat on the floor, toes pointed forward. Your torso is straight and perpendicular to the floor.

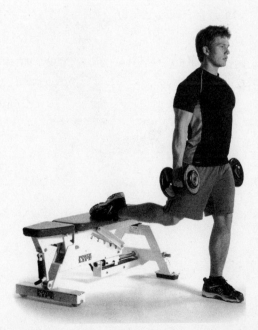

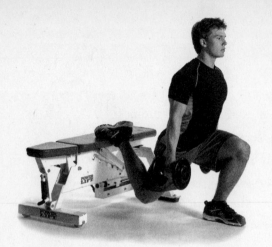

Lower your body until your left knee is bent at least 90 degrees and your right knee comes close to touching the floor. Your torso should remain upright. Push back up to the starting position, finish all your reps with your left leg, then switch and do the same number of reps with your right leg. That's one set.

Note: You can also do this holding a single dumbbell or weight plate with both hands in front of your chest.

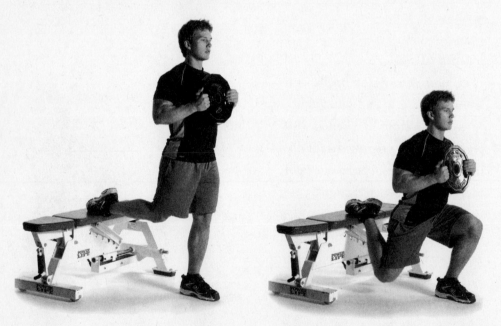

GOBLET SQUAT

The goods

You'll develop all your lower-body muscles, as you would with any squat variation. But, because you're holding the weight in front of your chest, you'll also improve your balance and core strength.

The gear

One dumbbell is all you need.

How to do it

Hold the dumbbell in front of you by cupping your hands under the top weight plates, as if you were going to drink out of it. With the weight touching your chest, set your feet slightly wider than your shoulders, toes pointed forward or angled out slightly. Tighten up your core.

Now push your hips back, descending as far as you can. Keep your elbows in line with your knees, rather than letting them flare out wider so they're outside your knees in the bottom position.

Push down through the middle of your feet to return to the starting position, and repeat.

THE GARAGE VARIATION: You can substitute a weight plate for the dumbbell.

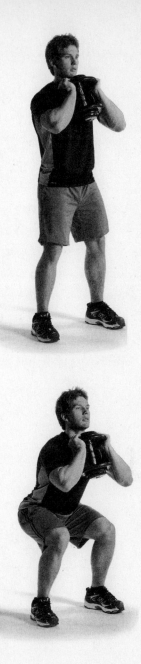

CABLE REVERSE WOOD CHOP

The goods/The gear

Same as for the cable wood chop (see page 122), except that you're using the low pulley instead of the high one.

How to do it

Attach the rope handle to the low pulley, and set yourself up sideways to the weight stack, with your right leg toward the machine. Stand with your feet shoulder-width apart, toes pointed forward, knees flexed slightly. Turn your shoulders to the right, reach down with both hands, and grab the rope attachment. As you did with the regular wood chop, turn your head with your shoulders so your eyes are on the rope.

Now pull the rope diagonally up and across your torso, rotating your shoulders as your hands end up above and to the outside of your left ear. Your eyes

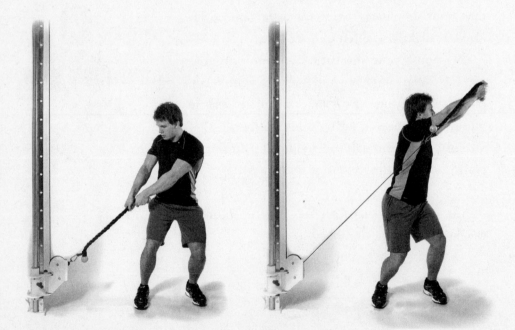

should follow the rope through the entire range of motion. As with the other exercise, your hips should face the same direction throughout the movement, keeping your lower back in a strong, stable position while your shoulders rotate. It's okay to pivot on the ball of your right foot, if that's a natural movement pattern for you.

Return to the starting position, finish your reps, then reverse your position and repeat the set.

THE GARAGE VARIATION: In contrast to the regular cable wood chop, there's a halfway decent version you can do without a cable. Just pull a dumbbell or medicine ball along the same diagonal trajectory. If you're using a medicine ball and have access to a really sturdy wall, you can actually let go of the ball at the top of the movement, slamming it against the wall and catching it as it bounces off.

SQUAT

The goods/The gear

Same as for the front squat (see page 114), except that this time the bar is on your back and you can use heavier weights.

How to do it

Set the bar in a power cage so it's at about shoulder level. Facing the bar, grab it with an overhand grip with your hands about one and a half times shoulder width. (It's the same grip you'd use for a barbell bench press.) Duck your head under the bar and squeeze your shoulder blades together in back, creating a shelf for the bar.

With the bar secure on your upper back, stand up, lifting the bar off the supports. Step back so your feet are shoulder-width apart and your toes are pointed forward or angled out slightly. Push your hips back and descend into a squat,

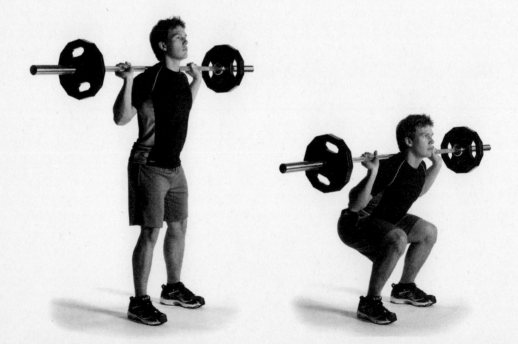

keeping your torso as upright as possible and your feet flat on the floor. Throughout the exercise, the bar should be directly over the middle of your feet, and your eyes should look straight ahead. (Don't look up toward the ceiling, no matter how many times you've seen powerlifters do it.)

Go down until your upper thighs are parallel to the floor, or as close as you can to that position while keeping your back in its natural arch.

Push down through your feet and rise to the starting position, making sure your lower back stays in the same position and your knees don't roll in or out.

Note: As you get tired toward the end of a set, you may notice that you're leaning farther forward, which means you're doing more of the work with your back and hips and less with your hips and thighs. That's the time to stop the set—don't keep doing reps when you can feel that your form has changed.

DUMBBELL ROMANIAN DEADLIFT

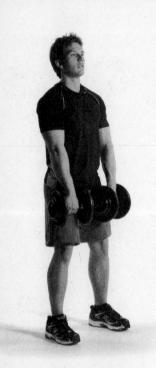

The goods

Here's another terrific exercise that focuses on your posterior chain—hamstrings, glutes, lower back.

The gear

Just dumbbells.

How to do it

Grab a pair of dumbbells with an overhand grip and stand holding them in front of your thighs with your feet shoulder-width apart (or slightly closer together, if you prefer), toes pointed straight ahead. Tighten your core.

Push your hips back as you lower the dumbbells until they're just past your knees. Keep your chest high and your lower back in its natural arch. Squeeze your glutes as you push your hips forward and return to the starting position.

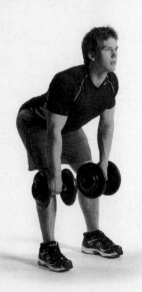

THE GARAGE VARIATION: You can also do this with a barbell, using an overhand grip that's just wider than your shoulders.

Note: This isn't a "stiff-legged" deadlift. Your knees will bend as much as they need to. The key is to start and finish the movement with your hips; your knees will take care of themselves.

REVERSE LUNGE

The goods

Lunges work all your lower-body muscles, while improving your balance and conditioning. I prefer to do these with a barbell, which raises the center of gravity and makes the exercise much tougher than it would be if you were holding dumbbells at your sides.

The gear

You'll need a barbell and a power cage.

How to do it

Set the barbell on supports at the same height you'd use for back squats and step-ups. Approach it backward, as you did for step-ups, and grab the bar with an overhand grip with your hands about one and a half times shoulder width. Squeeze your shoulder blades together, and rest the bar on the little shelf you create with your upper-back muscles. Lift the bar off the rack and take a step forward.

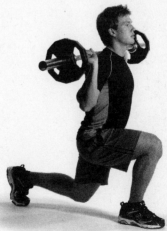

Stand with your feet hip-width apart, toes pointed forward. Take a long step back with your left leg, placing the ball of your foot on the floor. Drop down until your left knee almost touches the floor. Your torso should be upright, and your right shin perpendicular to the floor.

Step back to the starting position. Do all your reps stepping back with your left leg, then repeat with your right leg. That's one set.

THE GARAGE VARIATION: If you don't have a power cage, you'll have to lift the bar from the floor to your shoulders. If dumbbells are your only option, make the exercise harder by holding them up on your shoulders. You can hold them at the sides of your shoulders, as you would if you were doing shoulder presses, or tip them up and rest the dumbbells on your deltoids.

If you want to have even more fun, hold a single dumbbell overhead. Hold it in your left hand as you step back with your right leg, and vice versa.

BARBELL BENT-OVER ROW

The goods/The gear

Same as for the underhand version of the bent-over row (see page 126).

How to do it

Grab the bar with an overhand grip that's about one and a half times the width of your shoulders, or about the same place you'd hold a bar for bench presses. Set your feet shoulder-width apart, toes pointed forward, and hold the bar in front of your thighs.

Push your hips back as you fold your torso forward, keeping your midsection tight and your lower back in its natural arch. Your torso won't be parallel to the floor, but the angle of your torso relative to the floor should be 45 degrees or less. Pull the bar up to your lower chest, lower it until your arms are straight again, and repeat until you finish the set.

DON'T BE THAT GUY: As with any rowing exercise, you want the action in your shoulders, with your back and hips providing a solid base of support. The more you move that base, the less solid it is. So the best way to do bent-over rows, whether you're using barbells or dumbbells, is with your hips and torso in a fixed position.

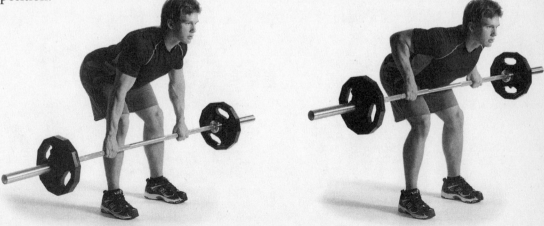

BARBELL INCLINE BENCH PRESS

The goods

Same as other bench-press variations.

The gear

You'll need an adjustable bench with uprights for the barbell.

How to do it

Set the incline bench so it's about 30 degrees relative to the floor. (You can go as high as 45 degrees or as low as 15 degrees.) Lie on your back on the bench and grab the bar with an overhand grip with your hands about one and a half times shoulder width. Set your feet wide and flat on the floor. Your lower back should be in its natural arch—not touching the bench.

Lift the bar off the uprights (it's a good idea to use a spotter for low-rep sets) and hold it over your upper chest with your arms straight. Lower the bar to your upper chest, then push the bar straight up to the starting position. Repeat to finish the set.

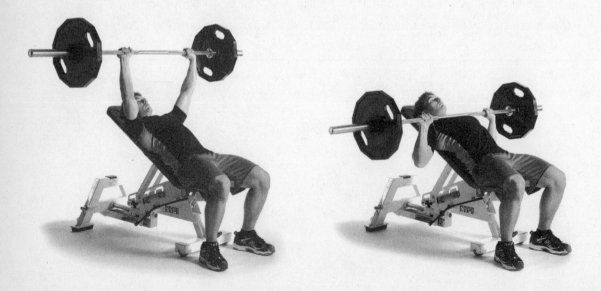

THE GARAGE VARIATION: Have I mentioned how much use you'll get out of a simple power cage? I've already described how to use it for lower-body exercises (squats, step-ups, and reverse lunges), chin-ups, and even dips if you buy a special attachment. I haven't mentioned that you can buy cable stations that attach to the back of your power cage, allowing you to do pulldowns and rows.

Now here's one more use: it's also perfect for barbell bench presses, including incline presses if you have an adjustable bench. Just slide your bench into the cage, set the uprights at an appropriate height for bench pressing, set the safety rails on the sides at a height that allows you to escape if you can't get the bar off your chest, and you're ready to go.

DUMBBELL SHOULDER PRESS

The goods/The gear

Same as for the shoulder press with neutral grip (see page 109).

How to do it

Grab a pair of dumbbells and stand with your feet shoulder-width apart, holding the weights just above and to the sides of your shoulders. Your thumbs are facing each other, with your knuckles toward the ceiling (overhand grip). Press the dumbbells straight up over your shoulders until your arms are straight. Keep your torso upright and your lower back in its natural arch—don't bow your back.

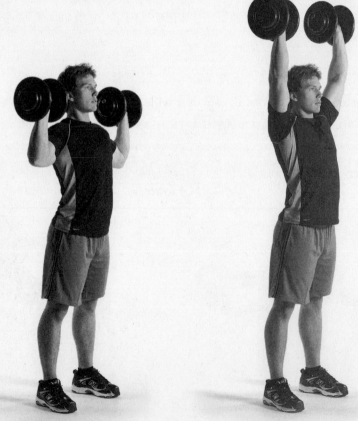

SWISS-BALL CRUNCH

The goods

This is a straightforward exercise directly targeting your rectus abdominis and obliques.

The gear

You'll need a Swiss ball (aka stability ball, balance ball, or physioball). The taller you are, the bigger the ball you need. If you're average height, between five feet seven and five feet eleven, you'll do fine with a 65-centimeter ball. (That's the diameter, obviously.) Shorter guys should opt for 55 centimeters. If you're over six feet, you'll need a 75-centimeter ball. And if you're over six-feet-three, you may need an 85-centimeter ball, which is rarely found in gyms unless they cater to NBA players.

How to do it

Sit on top of the ball with your feet wide apart and flat on the floor. Slide your hips forward until your lower back is centered atop the ball. Your knees should be bent about 90 degrees, with your thighs parallel to the floor. Touch your fingers to the sides of your head, just behind your ears. (Don't interlock them behind your head—it leads to bad form and might even strain your neck.) That's your starting position.

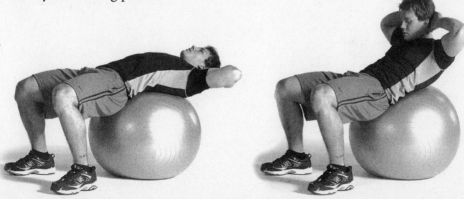

Now, keeping your hips and thighs up, crunch your abs to lift your shoulders and upper torso off the ball, rolling them toward your hips. Squeeze your abs at the top of the movement, then release and return to the starting position.

When it's easy to get all the designated reps, add resistance by holding a dumbbell or weight plate against your chest.

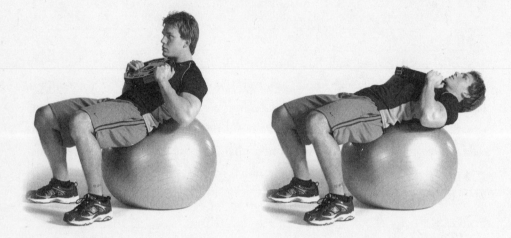

THE GARAGE VARIATION: Hey, break down and buy yourself a Swiss ball. Otherwise, you can make do with crunches on the floor, perhaps with a rolled towel beneath your lower back. Unless you're an absolute beginner, you'll probably need to use extra weight for resistance.

BARBELL PUSH PRESS

The goods

Since this is a shoulder press with momentum, you'll use heavier weights and more of your body's overall muscle mass. That means you'll develop greater strength and power, and probably burn more fat because of the higher degree of difficulty and greater exhaustion.

The gear

Just a barbell and a power cage that allows you to start with the barbell at shoulder level.

How to do it

Set the bar on the supports at chest level. Grab it overhand with your hands a bit wider than your shoulders. Lift it off the rack and step back, holding it across the front of your shoulders with your feet shoulder-width apart and toes pointed forward.

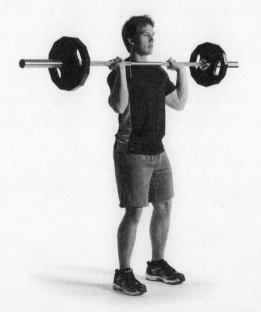

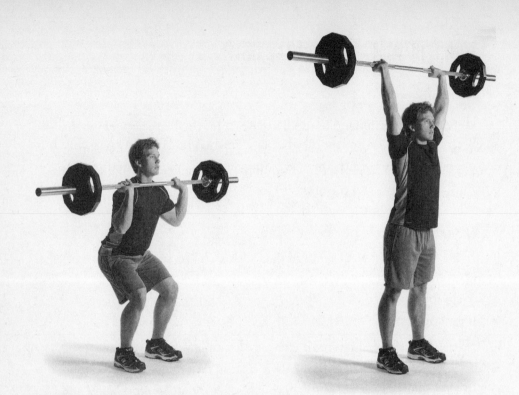

Push your hips back and dip down about a quarter of the distance you'd go down for a squat. Without pausing, push back up as powerfully as you can, using this momentum to drive the weight overhead. (You might come all the way up on your toes for the first reps of your set.) Finish the rep with straight legs and arms and the bar locked firmly overhead. Lower the weight quickly but under control, and immediately push your hips back for the next repetition.

THE GARAGE VARIATION: If you don't have a power cage, you'll have to start with the bar on the floor and lift it to your shoulders.

CABLE ROW WITH NEUTRAL GRIP

The goods

This uses the same upper-back muscles as other cable-row variations, but you'll use your arm muscles somewhat differently. You may not know this, but one of your most important upper-arm muscles is a thick, strong strip called the brachialis, which sits between the biceps and the upper-arm bone. It's hard to see unless your upper arms are already pretty well developed, but trust me, it's there, working hard to help your biceps bend your elbows on pulling exercises. Your biceps is in its strongest position when you use an underhand grip. In the neutral grip, the brachialis is in the stronger position. You'll be able to tell the first time you do this exercise—chances are you'll be able to work with more weight than you have on any other cable-row variation.

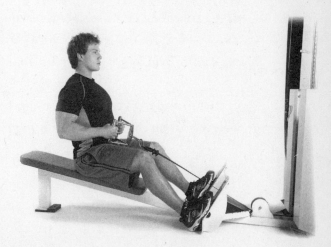

The gear

You'll need the triangle-shaped handle. If there isn't one near the cable-row station, chances are you'll find one at the lat-pulldown station.

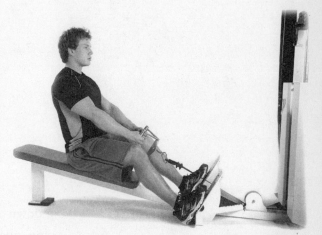

How to do it

Grab the triangle attachment with your palms facing each other, and set yourself up in the wide-grip cable row station (see page 100). Pull the handle to your abdomen, squeezing your shoulder blades together at the end of the movement. Return to the starting position and repeat.

Note: Remember back at the beginning of this chapter, when I mentioned that the cable-row station we used for these photos probably doesn't look exactly like the one you use at your gym? Well, here it is again.

DUMBBELL HANG SNATCH

The goods

This is a pure power move; you'll move as fast and explosively as possible, using your entire body and working up a serious sweat. It's great for body composition—more muscle (particularly in your upper back) with less fat—while also making your body faster and more athletic.

The gear

Just a single dumbbell.

How to do it

Hold the dumbbell with an overhand grip in your right hand, with your feet about hip-width apart (or slightly wider if that's more comfortable). Push your hips back and allow your knees to bend so your torso is bent forward and the dumbbell is between your legs and just below your knees. Keep your chest up and eyes facing forward. This is your starting position.

Now . . . jump. Your feet don't literally have to come off the floor, but your body should do what fitness geeks call "triple extension": your ankles, knees, and hips all straighten.

You're probably wondering what this has to do with the weight in your right hand. As you're coming up, you're going to pull the weight with your upper-back muscles. Don't consciously try to do anything with your arm muscles; just let your elbow bend naturally as the dumbbell comes up in front of your torso.

That brings you to the fun part: at the top of the "jump," when you're up on the balls of your feet and the dumbbell is at chest level, reverse the movement and drop your hips, while allowing the weight to continue upward until your arm is straight. Again, don't deliberately straighten your arm; just pull the weight hard enough at the beginning and drop down far enough at the end that your arm ends up straight over your head. Pause here, with your hips back and arm locked overhead.

Lower the weight to the starting position—you don't need to reverse your steps here, just let it drop with control. Finish all the reps with your right arm, then repeat with your left. That's one set.

Remember to do every repetition as fast and explosively as you can. All the action is in your posterior-chain muscles. The arm holding the weight is just along for the ride.

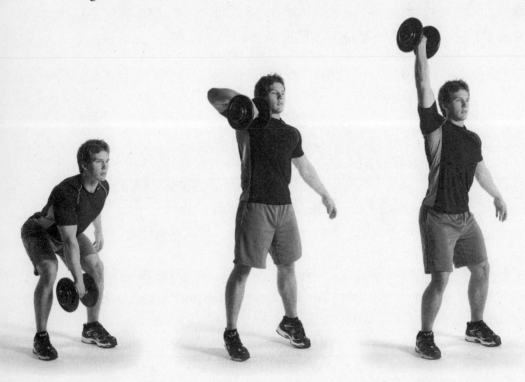

3-POINT PLANK

How to do it

This is the same as the plank (see page 112), except that you'll lift one foot off the floor. Start with your right, and switch legs every ten to fifteen seconds until you've held the plank for the designated amount of time. Make sure you do the same amount of work with each leg in the air.

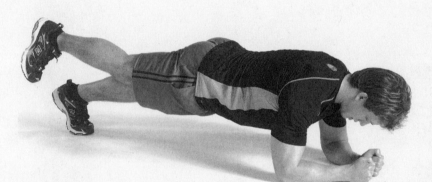

JUMP SQUAT

The goods

Although you're using the same muscles as in a regular squat, you're doing these for the metabolic benefit—you want to get your heart pounding and induce a level of fatigue that keeps your metabolism elevated long after you leave the gym.

The gear

Just your body weight.

How to do it

Set your feet shoulder-width apart, toes pointing forward. Put your hands behind your head, with fingers touching but not interlocked. Push your hips back as you descend into a squat; then without pausing jump straight up, point your toes, and catch a little air. Land on the balls of your feet to absorb the shock, then drop back onto your heels and immediately push your hips back to start the next repetition.

Try to do all your reps continuously and rhythmically.

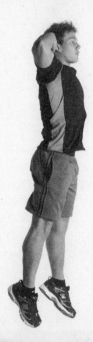

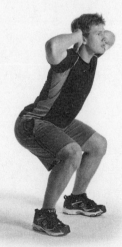

Note: When you feel confident that you've got the hang of the exercise, do it with an unloaded barbell on your back, then slowly progress to heavier weights.

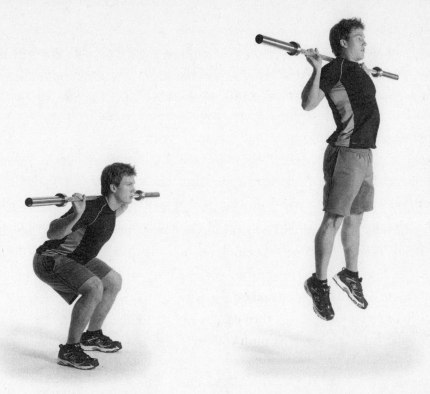

WIDE-GRIP PULL-UP

How to do it

Grab the pull-up bar with the widest overhand grip you can manage or that the bar allows. Hang with your arms straight and in the same plane as your torso and legs. (You can bend your knees and cross your ankles behind you, if you prefer.) Pull yourself up as high as you can, squeeze your upper-back muscles, then lower yourself with control and repeat.

Note: With some gym setups, the only handles that allow you to take a wide grip put your hands at a 45-degree angle, rather than a pure overhand grip. And if you're working out at home, your chin-up bar may not allow for a grip that's much wider than your shoulders. Either of those options is perfectly fine; focus on the exercise, not the details.

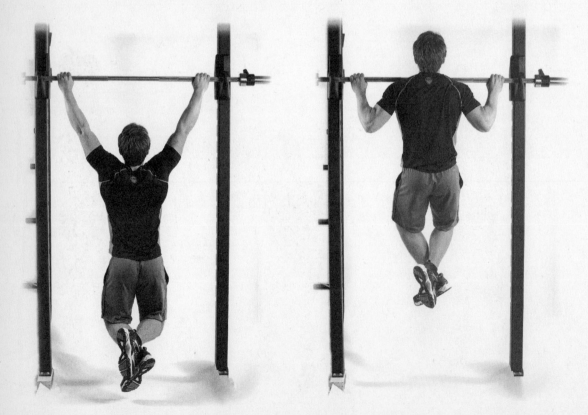

SINGLE-ARM PUSH PRESS

The goods

Same as the barbell push press (see page 153), only you're working with one arm at a time and thus doing twice as many reps per set.

The gear

Just a single dumbbell.

How to do it

Stand with your feet shoulder-width apart, holding a dumbbell in your left hand at the edge of your left shoulder, palm facing inward. Your nonworking

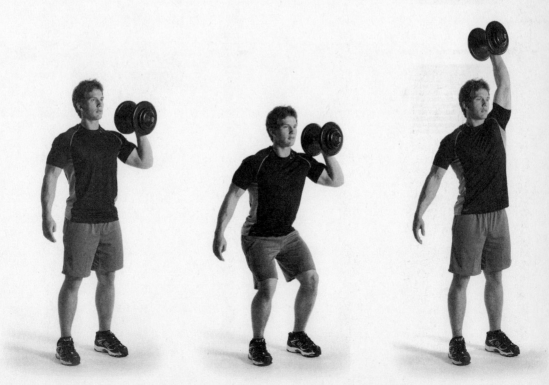

arm can be out to your side for balance. Dip your hips, then explode upward as you drive the dumbbell up until your arm is straight over your shoulder.

Come to a full stop with your arm locked overhead and legs straight, then lower the weight with control until it's back in the starting position. Immediately dip down to start the next repetition. Do all your reps with your left arm, then repeat with your right. That's one set.

BARBELL CLEAN PULL

The goods

This is a deadlift with a shoulder shrug, but done faster and with a lighter weight. It has all the benefits of the other explosive exercises I've described, with the addition of intense work for your traps. (Fair warning: They'll be sore—*really* sore—for the next two or three days.)

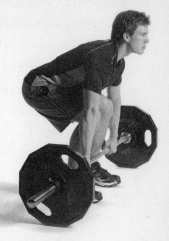

The gear

Just a barbell.

How to do it

Set up as you would for a deadlift (see page 135). Pull the bar up as fast as you can, but instead of stopping in the normal place, keep pulling by shrugging your shoulders and coming up onto the balls of your feet. Your arms stay straight throughout the movement, which is why this is such an intense challenge to your traps.

Relax your shoulders and come down off the balls of your feet. As soon as your heels hit the floor, immediately descend for the next rep. You don't have to make a complete stop with the bar on the floor; as soon as the plates make contact, start the next pull.

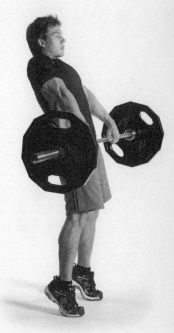

FRONT SQUAT TO PUSH PRESS

The goods

You get all the benefits of the two exercises in the title, along with a limit-testing level of exhaustion that will help keep your metabolism elevated for hours after you leave the gym, if not days.

The gear

Barbell and power cage.

How to do it

Set up as you would for the front squat (see page 114), with the bar resting on the front of your shoulders and held in place with your fingers. Your upper arms are parallel to the floor.

Push your hips back and descend into the front squat, then reverse your movement quickly and begin a powerful ascent.

As you're rising toward the starting position, roll the bar to your palms and drop your upper arms toward your torso. It takes a while to get the hang of it,

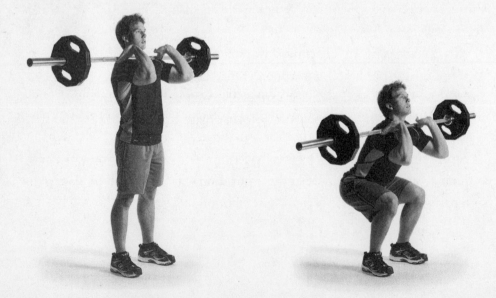

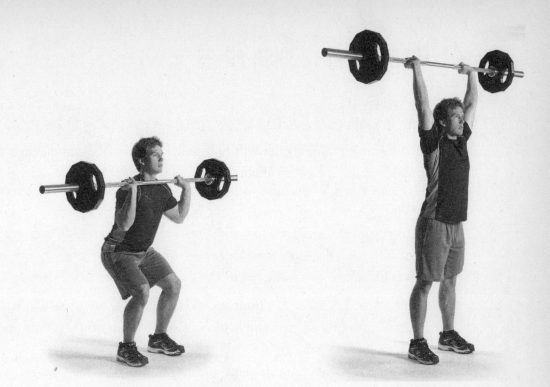

but eventually you can time this so you make a smooth transition to the push press (see page 153), and drive the barbell upward without having to think about when you should start pushing it.

You want to pause with the barbell locked overhead and your legs straight, as you did with the push press as a solo exercise.

Lower the bar to your shoulders, and roll it back from your palms to your fingertips until it rests on the front of your shoulders with your upper arms parallel to the floor. Immediately descend into the next front squat.

Again, this transition will eventually become so smooth that you won't have to think about resetting the weight on your shoulders, and you'll be able to do both parts of the exercise in a continuous motion.

JUMP LUNGE

How to do it

Start in a split stance, with your left leg in front and your right leg back. Your left foot is flat, while the ball of your right foot is on the floor. Hold your hands behind your head, with your fingers touching but not interlocked.

Drop down into a lunge position, with your left knee bent about 90 degrees and your right knee nearly touching the floor. Now jump as high as you can, switching feet in midair so you land with your right leg forward and left leg back. Immediately descend into the next lunge and repeat the jump. That's one rep.

Note: Once you get proficient in the movements, add weight by holding dumbbells at your sides.

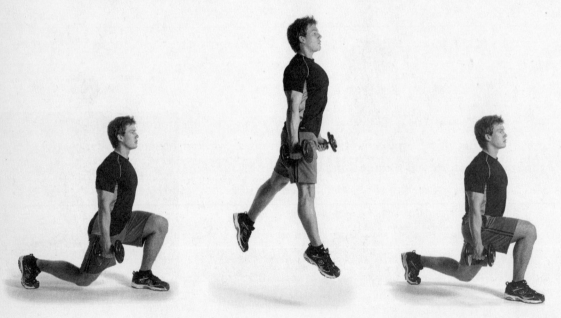

BULGARIAN SPLIT SQUAT, FRONT FOOT ELEVATED

How to do it

This is the second-most-hated exercise in my studio. It's exactly the same as the most-hated exercise, the Bulgarian split squat (see page 137), only harder. (My clients would hate it more if they knew it was coming. By the time they get to it, they've used up all their best hate on the original exercise.)

Start with your front foot elevated on a low step or box. (You can also use a forty-five-pound weight plate laid flat on the floor.) The extra height of your front foot increases the range of motion, which makes the exercise even tougher.

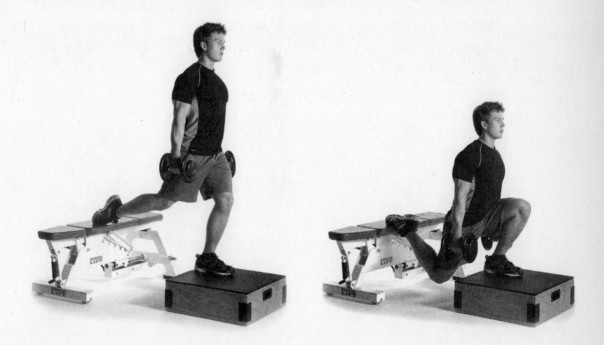

PUSH-UP

The goods

If you think push-ups are easy, you probably aren't doing them right. Done properly, they challenge your core muscles along with your chest, shoulders, and triceps. Because your body weight is resting on your hands and toes, you're pushing about 60 percent of your weight on each repetition. So you won't build strength and muscle mass the way you can with heavy-duty bench presses. But if you keep your body in the correct alignment, you'll develop enough core strength and endurance to make up for it.

Here's the bottom line: unless you're bench-pressing your partner instead of having sex with her, the most popular chest-building exercise has no direct correlation with your lovemaking skill. But the push-up is something else entirely: you don't have to strain your imagination to think of the many ways in which core strength comes in handy in the bedroom, especially when it's combined with an ability to support your own weight with your upper-body muscles.

The gear

Just the floor and you.

How to do it

Get into push-up position, with your hands directly beneath your shoulders and your weight resting on your palms and toes. Your body should form a straight line from neck to ankles. Lower your chest until it's an inch or two from

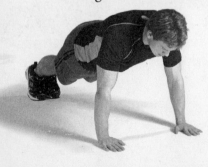 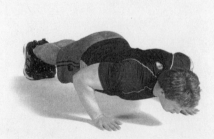

the floor, and then push up to the starting position. Keep your body in the same alignment throughout.

ROCK-CLIMBER PUSH-UP

The goods

You can think up any number of ways to make push-ups more challenging—you can elevate your feet off the floor, you can move your hands in closer together, you can put your hands on a medicine ball or Swiss ball . . . really, you're only limited by your imagination.

This push-up is one of my favorites, if for no other reason than because of the looks I get if I do these in a public place. If you do any rock climbing or high-level tree-hugging, this exercise has functional benefits as well.

The gear

Just the floor and you.

How to do it

Get into a push-up position. As you lower your body, bend your right leg and rotate your right knee outward until it's outside your right elbow. Don't drag your foot, and try not to allow your torso to rotate. Return to the starting position and repeat, pulling your left knee to your left elbow.

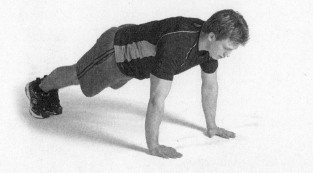 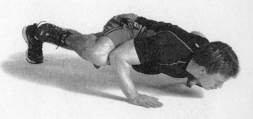

LAT PULLDOWN WITH NEUTRAL GRIP

The goods

You're using basically the same back muscles that you use on other variations of the lat pulldown, with two interesting differences. Because your arms are close together in front of your chest, you end up using your pecs more than you would in other pulldown variations. And instead of using your biceps in a direct line of pull, as you do in the underhand-grip pulldown, you emphasize a thick muscle called the brachialis, described earlier with the neutral-grip cable row (see page 155).

Since this is the most biomechanically advantageous hand and arm position, you'll be able to pull heavier weights than on other pulldown variations. The combination of heavier weights and bonus muscle involvement from your pecs and brachialis makes this a really good exercise for thickening your arms and upper torso.

The gear

You'll need the triangle-shaped handle for the lat-pulldown station.

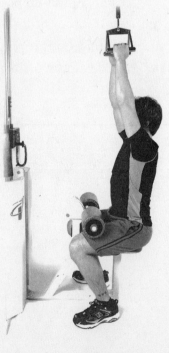

How to do it

Grab the triangle attachment with your palms facing each other, and set yourself up in the lat-pulldown station (see page 107). Pull the handle down to the top of your chest, squeezing your shoulder blades together at the end of the movement. Return to the starting position and repeat.

THE GARAGE VARIATION: There's really no perfect imitation you can do at home if you don't have a lat-pulldown apparatus. But there are some good exercises you can do instead. One is the reverse push-up, aka horizontal chin-up (see page 107). Use an overhand grip in which your hands are close together, with your thumbs perhaps six inches apart. You can also try that close hand position on a barbell bent-over row.

Note: It's actually okay to lean back more than on other lat-pulldown variations. Just make sure your torso remains at the same angle throughout the range of motion.

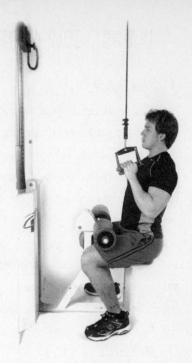

BARBELL REVERSE CURL

The goods

Yes, finally, you get to do a biceps curl. But it's not the kind you really want to do. I just described how the brachialis comes into play on the neutral-grip lat pulldown. On the reverse curl, the brachialis's partner, a forearm muscle called the brachioradialis, gets the best workout. The brachialis also works hard here, but the biceps are in their weakest possible position.

The gear

You can use either a straight barbell or an EZ-curl bar—it's the barbell with the zigzag shape in the middle, allowing you to use hand positions that are in between overhand and underhand.

How to do it

Grab the barbell overhand with a grip that's about shoulder width. Stand holding the bar in front of your thighs. Keeping your upper arms at your sides

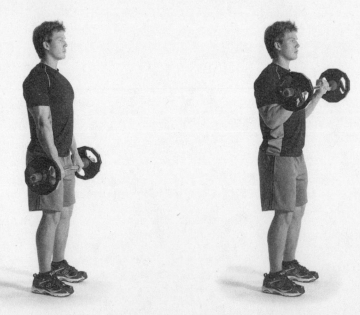

and moving only your elbows, curl the bar straight up to your chest. Squeeze your arm muscles at the top, then lower the bar and repeat.

Note: I could go apeshit here with all my admonitions to keep your form as strict as possible. But nobody does curls with perfect form—there's always some movement at the shoulders, and most of us lean back slightly with our torsos, particularly toward the end of the set. (And of course there's movement in the wrist joints.) So my advice here is to use common sense. If you find yourself rocking and swaying with every rep, you're using too much weight. But a little body movement isn't the end of the world.

DUMBBELL ALTERNATING CURL

The goods

Now you're targeting your biceps directly, with your brachialis and brachio-radialis in supporting roles. This is one exercise where slightly loose form is actually beneficial. If your front arm comes forward a bit more than it would on a barbell biceps curl, that's fine, because it incorporates shoulder muscles. Also, because you're alternating arms, you're shifting your balance and creating a mild challenge for your core muscles. I'm not suggesting that you go nuts and invent a whole new exercise here. I just want to point out that extra movements do incorporate extra muscles, and that's not always a bad thing.

The gear

Two dumbbells.

How to do it

Grab a pair of dumbbells and let them hang to your sides with your palms facing in, arms straight. Starting with your left side if you're right-handed, and

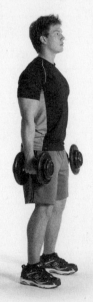 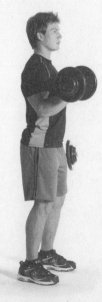

your right side if you're a lefty, bend your left elbow and curl the dumbbell up toward your left shoulder, rotating your forearm on the way up so your left palm faces the front of your shoulder at the top. Squeeze your biceps, then lower the dumbbell, rotating it back to the original position.

When it's near the bottom, begin curling the weight in your right hand. Continue alternating to complete the set, doing the designated number of reps with each arm.

DUMBBELL INCLINE BENCH PRESS WITH NEUTRAL GRIP

How to do it

Follow the directions for the dumbbell incline bench press (see page 128), only using a neutral grip—your palms facing each other.

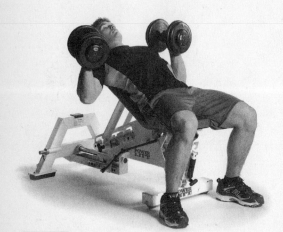

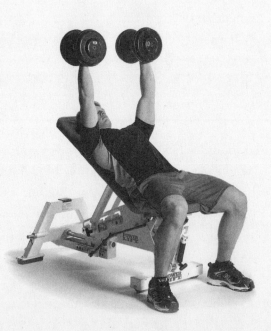

DUMBBELL LYING TRICEPS EXTENSION

The goods

This exercise hits your triceps directly, if not as forcefully as you hit them on dips and presses.

The gear

Two dumbbells and a flat bench.

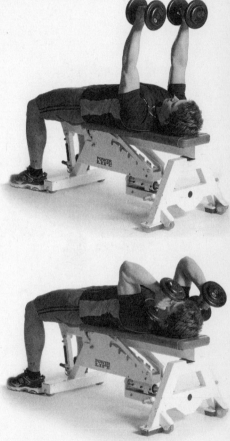

How to do it

Grab two dumbbells and lie on your back on a flat bench, with your legs wide and feet on the floor. With your arms straight, hold the weights over your face, with your palms facing each other. Now, moving only at the elbows (keep this movement stricter than your biceps curls), lower the weights until they're down by your ears. Straighten your arms to return them to the starting position, and repeat.

THE GARAGE VARIATION: If you don't have two matching dumbbells, you can do this with a single dumbbell by cupping your hands beneath the weight plates at the top end of the dumbbell. I know that sounds confusing as shit, but it's really pretty simple: if you stand a dumbbell up on one end, you want to put your hands beneath the weight plates on the top end. Then do the exercise as described.

You can also do the same thing with an EZ-curl bar or straight barbell, using an overhand grip that's about shoulder width.

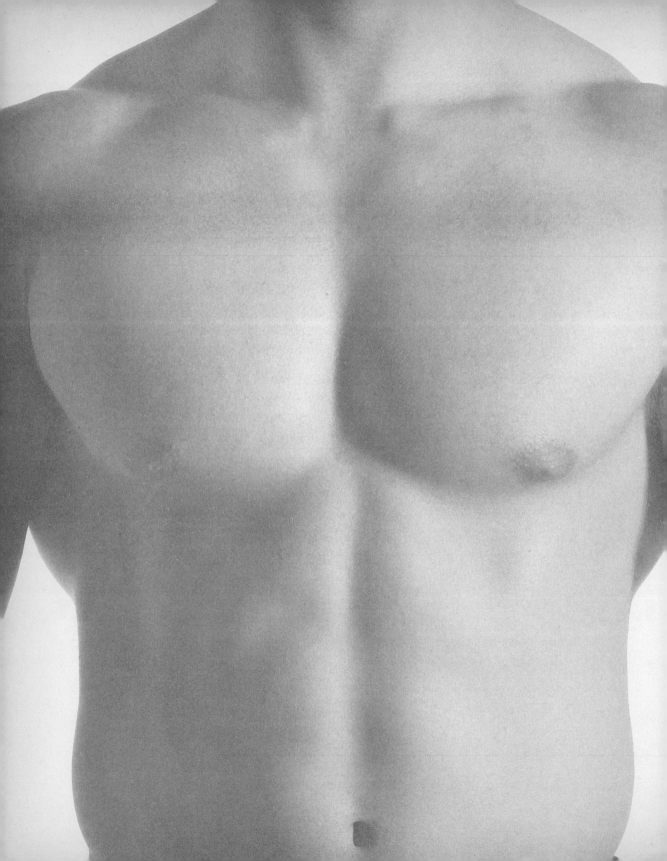

PART 3

Feeding, Clothing, and
Showing Off the Body
You've Built

CHAPTER NINE

These Foods Can Make or Break Your Physique

I know, I know. You didn't buy this book to learn my special recipe for grilled pork tenderloin, and you certainly don't want to talk about the ideal mix of protein, carbohydrates, and fat in your diet when chances are that your diet consists of whatever you can find in five minutes or less. If the nearest available food carries a low risk of salmonella poisoning, that's even better.

I could give you a long grocery list and tell you what to eat at every meal for the next year, but it wouldn't be much help if your bank has been forced to pry your credit cards from your cold, dead wallet.

Cooking? Yeah, right. If a guy wants to spend more quality time with his saucepans, he knows better than to look for that kind of information in a book like this (although I do have some quick and easy recipes at builtforshow.com). Sure, culinary skill comes in handy when you've invited a date over for a home-cooked dinner; I don't need to explain why boiling dinosaur-shaped mac 'n' cheese right out of the box doesn't count as "cooking" to the modern female of our species. (It also doesn't count as "dinner" for either you or your date, although I'm getting ahead of myself here.) But we both know I'm not the guy to teach you such skills.

We also know that very few guys have the time, energy, or cash flow to eat right every day, at every meal. And even if such a thing were possible, most of us wouldn't want to. What's the point of being young if you can't do stupid shit to your body every now and then? You need something to remember fondly when you're old and have actual responsibilities.

Still, I'd be doing you no favors if I blew off the subject of nutrition entirely. What you eat, and how you eat it, is at least as important as what you lift and how you lift it. You can't be built for show if your diet blows. So we have to boil this conversation down to its essence—to the basic framework of a healthy, muscle-friendly, body-fat-averse diet—without getting bogged down in the details.

You can eat better than you're eating now without going broke, without spending any more time in the kitchen than you want to, without restricting your diet to chicken breasts and broccoli, and without having to carry a calculator with you everywhere you go to count calories. This ain't Jenny Craig.

WHAT IS "HEALTHY" FOOD?

Let's start with a sweeping generalization. It's by no means original (if I could remember where I heard it I'd be happy to give credit where it's due), but I think it's a useful starting point: If your grandparents and great-grandparents would've recognized it as "food," it's probably good for you. Or, at worst, not particularly bad for you.

You could include any type of meat or fish, eggs, dairy products, fruits and vegetables, and fresh-baked bread.

But there's a problem with this generalization. Your great-grandparents could've walked into a butcher shop and bought sausages of any shape and description, filled with who knows what. (They weren't sticklers for nutrition labels back then.) They would've baked or bought pies with crusts made with lard.

The fresh milk that was delivered to their front door came with super-high-fat cream that had risen to the top of the bottle. And they fried damn near everything. None of those things will kill you fast, or even be particularly bad for your long-term health as an occasional indulgence, but if you want to be built for show, you need to keep the piecrust and fried anything to a minimum.

So let's try a stricter definition.

If you went back ten thousand years in human history, before there was such a thing as agriculture (or history, now that I think about it), just about anything our ancestors might have hunted, caught, dug up, or gathered would probably be considered good for you by today's standards. The meat was lean (slow, blubbery animals didn't last long in the wild), the fish were untainted with mercury, the eggs would've come straight out of a pissed-off bird or tortoise's nest, and you wouldn't have had to worry about pesticides on the roots and berries.

But the most important difference is that there was no such thing as processed food. They might've ground up seeds and grains, or figured out that boiled roots are a lot easier on your teeth than when they're raw. But, for the most part, people back then had to eat food that was pretty close to the way they'd found it. A balanced diet was eating the brains of an animal they'd killed, along with the meat.

So let's say that's the ideal (aside from the "eating brains" part). But let's also concede that, as guidelines go, "eat like a caveman" isn't particularly helpful.

Where does that leave us?

Every nutritional expert has his or her own set of guidelines about what a "healthy" diet should include. Here's my take:

Red Meat

BENEFITS: Lots of high-quality protein, some healthy fats; satisfies your appetite; provides a need for the dental-floss industry to exist.

DRAWBACKS: Most meat that comes from hoofed animals (especially the type of meat you and I can afford) has been fattened up with grain, reducing its nutritional quality; you might also get hormones and antibiotics in the meat, and perhaps even pesticides from the animals' feed.

TYPES TO AVOID MOST OF THE TIME: Fast-food burgers; hot dogs; frozen breakfast sausages made from pork.

OKAY CHOICES: Round steak (T-bone, if your dad or your boss is paying); cheapest store-bought hamburger; burgers in sit-down restaurants (the kind with menus).

GOOD CHOICES: Ground sirloin (the package will say "90 percent lean") or any type of pork or beef that includes "loin" in the name.

REALLY GOOD CHOICES THAT MOST OF US CAN'T AFFORD: Pasture-raised beef, from animals allowed to graze on natural grasses throughout their lives—it'll have higher levels of healthy fats, like those found in fish.

Things with wings

BENEFITS: Mostly the same as for other meat—lots of muscle-friendly protein; white meat tends to be leaner than even the leanest types of red meat; hard to eat too much, because the flavor is kind of boring (chicken, after all, tastes like chicken).

DRAWBACKS: Mediocre flavor; risk of food poisoning if poultry is undercooked.

TYPES TO AVOID MOST OF THE TIME: Whatever comes in a box at a fast-food restaurant with a container of honey-mustard sauce on the side; anything fried; whatever your mom defrosted for you when she was too tired to cook.

OKAY CHOICES: Dark meat of chicken or turkey, minus the skin (which has too much fat to be worth the boost in flavor); lower-fat versions of frozen chicken nuggets; fried chicken with the fried part (the skin) removed.

GOOD CHOICES: Baked or grilled chicken breast; white meat of turkey.

REALLY GOOD CHOICES THAT MOST OF US CAN'T AFFORD: Free-range birds, the type you might buy at a local farmers' market, which haven't been stuffed with grain and juiced with hormones; duck, which is higher in fat but a lot tastier than chicken or turkey.

Fish

BENEFITS: More high-quality protein; healthiest fats on the planet.

DRAWBACKS: High-quality fish is expensive; fish is relatively difficult to prepare; fresh fish doesn't last more than a day or two in the fridge; "predator" fish like shark or tuna may have high levels of mercury.

TYPES TO AVOID MOST OF THE TIME: Anything that smells fishy or is slimy to the touch; the fried fish they sell in the church basement on Friday nights; anything sold by a fast-food restaurant that has "Mc" in the front and/or "wich" at the end.

OKAY CHOICES: Tuna or salmon chunks that come in a can or pouch; some frozen fish you can defrost at home (check the nutrition labels to see how much fat and protein it has).

GOOD CHOICES: Baked or grilled fish, especially salmon (it has lots of healthy fats with very low risk of mercury, since it's not a predator).

REALLY GOOD CHOICES THAT MOST OF US CAN'T AFFORD: Lots of guys will say they don't like fish, but let me tell you: once you've had a salmon entrée in a high-end restaurant, cooked when it's fresh by a professional chef, you'll never say you don't like fish again.

Dairy and eggs

BENEFITS: Highest-quality protein on the planet; low price; eggs last a long time in your fridge; dairy has calcium, which helps your muscles work better and may have a role in making you leaner; eggs are easy to prepare, even for guys like us.

DRAWBACKS: None, really, other than the fact that milk can go bad (especially if you forget to put it back in the fridge) and eggs can't be eaten raw without some risk of food poisoning.

TYPES TO AVOID MOST OF THE TIME: "Whole" milk or cream (including the cream you get in high-calorie coffees at Starbucks); yogurt with more than 15 grams of sugar per serving; margarine (not technically a dairy product, but it's sold with them); American cheese; cream cheese.

OKAY CHOICES: "Fruit on the bottom" yogurt; butter (it's all fat, but some of the fats are the healthiest types); cheddar and other types of hard cheese.

GOOD CHOICES: Eggs cooked just about any way you like them (other than fried in bacon fat); nonfat (skim) or 2 percent milk; mozzarella cheese (including string cheese); unflavored yogurt.

REALLY GOOD CHOICE THAT MOST OF US CAN'T LOOK AT WITHOUT GAGGING: Cottage cheese gives you the best concentration of milk proteins and calcium that you'll find without using a whey-protein supplement.

Fruits and vegetables

BENEFITS: Whatever your mom told you is probably true—great sources of vitamins and minerals, and the fiber helps you feel fuller longer between meals; for fruits, prep is minimal, unless your schedule is so tight you can't find time to peel an orange; most veggies can be eaten raw or cooked; the protein in beans and some other veggies isn't the best type for building muscle, but it's better than no protein.

DRAWBACKS: Fresh fruit doesn't stay "fresh" for long (and I say that as the proud owner of more than my share of brown bananas); lettuce wilts even faster; some veggies are tricky to cook without overcooking.

TYPES TO AVOID MOST OF THE TIME: Iceberg lettuce (no nutritional value whatsoever); anything that violates the sensitivity of your taste buds, like beets or Brussels sprouts (both of which are good choices if you like them); anything that you feel compelled to dump nutritionally worthless salad dressing over before you can stand to eat it.

OKAY CHOICES: Higher-calorie, low-fiber, lower-nutrient choices like bananas and potatoes.

GOOD CHOICES: Generally, the deeper the color of the fruit or vegetable, the better it is; the more colors you eat in a day or a week, the greater the variety of vitamins and minerals you'll take in; colors include orange and yellow (carrots, oranges, squash), red (tomatoes, watermelon), and green (spinach, lettuce, broccoli).

REALLY GOOD CHOICES THAT MOST OF US CAN'T AFFORD: Most of us will grow into adulthood without ever knowing how good spinach and other high-yuck-factor vegetables can taste when prepared by a good chef in an expensive restaurant.

Grains, cereals, breads

BENEFITS: If you're trying to gain weight, or just maintain your weight while doing a serious workout program, grains offer lots of calories at a low price; unless you're into homemade bread, these are some of the easiest foods to prepare; most of them taste okay.

DRAWBACKS: Easy to eat too much if you're struggling with weight control; if it comes in a box, it's probably not good for you, since all the good stuff has been taken out and lots of questionable stuff has been put in for flavor and texture.

TYPES TO AVOID MOST OF THE TIME: Chips and other high-salt, low-nutrition snack foods; high-sugar, low-fiber breakfast cereals, especially the ones they market to children on Saturday morning TV shows; anything that falls into the "pastry" category, like muffins, doughnuts, scones, cookies, cake, croissants, scones; white bread, including most bagels; instant microwave oatmeal, since it's much lower in fiber and much higher in sugar than slower-cooking oatmeal; breakfast bars.

OKAY CHOICES: Whole-grain bread, including whole-grain bagels or English muffins; low-sugar breakfast cereals like Cheerios; white rice and regular pasta.

GOOD CHOICES: Cereals that are high in fiber and whole grains, like Kashi and All-Bran; slow-cooked oatmeal (usually called "rolled oats" on the label); brown rice; long-grain wild rice (which is really a type of grass seed); whole-grain pasta.

REALLY GOOD CHOICE THAT MOST OF US WOULD NEVER CONSIDER: If you make your own bread, which isn't all that difficult with an electric bread maker, you can keep it simple with whole wheat flour and virtually none of the crap that commercial bakeries put into their packaged breads to make them softer, tastier, and longer-lasting on store shelves. It takes a bit of cash to buy the bread-making machine and a small investment of time, energy, and money to shop for the ingredients and make the bread, and those are deal-breakers for most of us. But the bread that results is really, really good, especially that first slice that you have when the bread's still hot out of the machine.

Condiments

I won't bother with the whole "benefits versus drawbacks," "good choices versus bad choices" thing here. A general drawback of eating healthier food, especially salads and vegetables, is that you're tempted to dump craploads of condiments on top of them. You can say the same thing about the cheapest hamburger: the lower the quality, and the faster it's prepared, the more gunk you'll want to add to give it some flavor.

You could even throw hamburger and hot dog buns into the category of condiments, since the ones with the least nutritional value tend to be the tastiest. The tastier the bun, and the more condiments you throw onto it, the easier it is to choke down whatever it is you've wrapped the bun around.

Most condiments, in small quantities, are okay. Ketchup and mustard have hardly any calories. But when you start spooning mayonnaise onto your sandwiches, there's a problem. Mayonnaise is made from soybean oil, the main component of which is a type of fat that you already get way too much of in meat and other condiments, especially salad dressings. (You probably don't eat a lot of salads, but the basic salad-dressing formula turns up in all kinds of fast foods.) It's also in lots of prepared foods, like muffins. A little isn't bad for you by any stretch, but a lot of it screws with your body's natural need to balance different types of fats.

Olive oil is a much better choice. It's a type of fat your body can use easily for energy, and it adds flavor to sandwiches and salads. Butter is also a decent choice, as I mentioned in the "Dairy and Eggs" section. It has a range of fats, including some that make your body stronger at the cellular level.

Another surprising way to make just about anything taste better is to add some nuts, like cashews, sunflower seeds, almonds, or pecans.

PUTTING A MEAL PLAN TOGETHER

Part 1. What to eat, generally

You could sum up everything in the previous section pretty simply: Eat lean meat, and fish and poultry, eggs, milk, fruits, vegetables, whole-grain breads and cereals, and nuts. Avoid ready-to-eat stuff that comes in a box or a vacuum-sealed bag whenever possible.

When all else fails, read the nutrition labels before you buy something in a grocery store. Some parts of labels are easy to figure out—I'll explain in a moment—while others are deliberately mysterious. You practically need a degree in nutritional biochemistry to understand all the words on labels. I'm in the fitness industry, and I don't know what a lot of that stuff is.

The easiest way to use a label is to look at the list of ingredients. The first thing on the list should be what you think you're buying. If it's a bread or cereal product, for example, the first ingredient should include the words "whole grain," or something to that effect. If it lists "enriched" flour first, that means it's not made from whole grains. Once you get beyond the first item on the list of ingredients, labels can be confusing, but I'll try to help you decipher some key points.

The main part of the label tells you how many calories the product has per serving, and breaks down the type of calories to a limited extent. The easiest call is on protein; the more you see, the better a choice it probably is.

Labels also tell you how much fat something has, plus the amount of saturated and trans fats, even if those numbers are both zero. Everyone knows trans fats are bad for you, so manufacturers figured out how to take them out of food without necessarily adding back anything that's good for you. Saturated fat is also broken down on labels, which prompted the food industry to start limiting it, but again, knowing something is low in saturated fat doesn't tell you much unless you know what's in there instead. If it's soybean oil (the main ingredient in mayonnaise, as I mentioned earlier), an absence of saturated fat isn't doing you any favors.

They also break down carbohydrates a bit, telling you how much sugar and fiber something has. Fiber, like protein, is an easy call; if two products are otherwise equal to the best of your judgment, the one with more fiber is probably better.

Sugar is a more difficult call. If you're pretty sure it's added sugar (the list of ingredients will probably include "corn syrup" or "high-fructose corn syrup"), then you can guess the product is pretty sucky. But if it's not a lot of sugar—a couple of grams—and the ingredients appear way down on the list, it's not a deal-breaker.

Breads and cereals—or anything made from grains—can have a lot of carbohydrates without having any added sugar. By contrast, just about all the carbs in fruit come from sugar, which is natural. Is an apple worse for you than a slice of bread? Of course not. But that's the problem with judging something by sugar alone.

One final note about labels: the line that tells you "calories per serving" can be surprisingly helpful. Let's say you're having a cookout and you're trying to decide what kind of hot dog or hamburger buns to buy. The "serving size" is always one bun—nobody eats a burger with three-quarters of a bun, or one and a half buns. Almost everybody at your barbecue, including you, is going to eat an entire bun with every burger or dog. So if one bun has 120 calories, and another has 150, that's a small but real difference. If you're trying to get leaner for summer, and figure you'll eat two burgers at your own cookout, that's 60 calories just from the buns, before you cut back on anything else that might make a difference to your waistline.

Part 2. When to eat, generally

I really have only two inviolable rules of nutrition for the guy who wants to be built for show:

1. Eat breakfast every single day.
2. Eat a postworkout meal immediately after lifting.

Words alone don't do justice to the importance of these two rules. I could put them in the biggest, boldest typeface, and I'm not sure it would be enough. If I could add sound effects—trumpets blaring, heavenly hosts proclaiming—I would.

There's no fast, foolproof way to reach your goals here. For each guy, it's going to be a little different. But if I've learned anything from my own experience and that of my clients, it's that people who follow the two inviolable rules get results faster than people who don't.

Let's take the rules one at a time.

WHY BREAKFAST IS NONNEGOTIABLE

Ever since elementary school, you've been told that "breakfast is the most important meal of the day." Yeah, I know you were told lots of things in elementary school that weren't remotely true (like "Bullies are unhappy people who're secretly jealous of you"; chances are, the guy who took your lunch money in sixth grade is now in management, where he's perfectly happy because he gets to bully people without having to get his knuckles dirty), but this is one thing our parents and teachers got right.

Muscle grows and fat goes when our metabolisms are revved up and we have a steady stream of nutrients circulating through our bodies. It takes calories to digest calories, which is why eating speeds up your metabolism. Eating at the right times pushes that food into the right places, like your muscles, and keeps it out of the wrong places, like the flesh that hangs over your belt.

If you're sleeping eight hours a night, as I described in Chapter 3 (if you're not, you should be), that's one-third of the day with no food. Most of us go to bed a couple hours after our last meal, so that means a fast of ten hours, or 42 percent of the day. If you also wait a couple hours after waking up to have breakfast, you're spending 50 percent of your day with a slower metabolism and without the nutrients you can use to build and repair your muscles.

I won't get into the technical details of why your body is most receptive to food when you first wake up. (If I did, I'd have to pretend that I *understand* those technical details, which would be funny, but not in a good way.) But I will say that your body needs and wants to replenish its supply of blood sugar after eight to ten hours without food, and your body's hormones are primed to use that food.

If you ignore my advice, and all the advice you've gotten since you were out of diapers, your body will go the other direction: hormones that prevent muscle building will suppress the ones that make it possible. Don't kid yourself into thinking that you can save a few calories and get leaner by skipping breakfast.

We have a label for people like that. We call them "fat people." Starving your body in the morning is a pretty good guarantee that you'll compensate later in the day by overfeeding.

Final point about breakfast: if you were to create the perfect diet for putting fat on your body, you'd skip breakfast and eat almost all your daily calories in a single meal. How do I know? Because that's the traditional way sumo wrestlers eat. That's how you create elite athletes who happen to weigh as much as six hundred pounds.

Sumo wrestlers do it because it's their profession, and from what I hear it's a great way to get laid in certain parts of the world. For you and me, the less we resemble sumo champions, the better our chances for hooking up.

WHY YOU NEED TO EAT AFTER YOUR WORKOUT

You can spend a lifetime working out and observing the things other people do when they work out, and you'll always find new reasons to confirm one of your darkest suspicions: hardly anybody knows what the hell he's doing.

But you have to give credit where it's due, and a lot of muscleheads in a lot of gyms deserve props for getting at least one thing right. They know they're supposed to have a protein shake immediately after their workouts. It helps explain why some guys with really bad workout programs can have really good bodies.

I should say here, before I go any further, that the best postworkout shake in the world won't make up for a half-assed workout. I should also note that protein shakes, with or without good workouts, won't override the cumulative effects of bad nutrition and/or poor sleep habits throughout the week. And, just for the sake of completeness, I should add that a great workout system combined with great nutrition and lifestyle choices can leave you with a great physique, even if you skip the postworkout shake.

So my point isn't that postworkout protein shakes are magic. You could probably accomplish the same thing with a regular meal immediately after you finish lifting. Shakes are just easier and more convenient to use, and don't leave anything to chance. You know you're getting protein and carbs in the most easily digestible form exactly when your body can make the best use of those things.

Why the urgency?

Well, let's remember that during a workout, you aren't really building muscle. You're tearing it apart. I mentioned earlier that all your body's tissues are constantly replenishing themselves. That's especially true for your muscles. Your body is always breaking down muscle protein, and then adding new protein to replace it. Lifting heavy weights in a systematic way accelerates this process. In fact, it's the *entire point* of lifting heavy weights in a systematic way. But lifting, by itself, only accelerates the "breaking down muscle protein" part of the equation. If you want to accelerate the part where your body adds new muscle protein, you have to give it some protein to work with. The faster you do this, the better.

You add carbs to that shake for two reasons: first, because your muscles need to replace the blood sugar that you've used for energy in your workout, and second, because the combination of protein and carbs should make the process go faster.

Need an analogy? Think of your postworkout shake as an elite special forces team armed with supplies (nutrients) that's been sent to rescue its comrades (damaged muscle tissue) from behind enemy lines.

Part 3. What to eat, specifically

BREAKFAST

A good breakfast will have a combination of slow-burning carbohydrates and fast-acting protein. Pick one option from each of the following lists to create your own breakfast. Feel free to mix and match all you want. Each option will take approximately five to seven minutes to prepare. (Really. Time yourself if you don't believe me.)

Staples
- Eggs (scrambled is easiest)
- Oatmeal (rolled oats are best; Weight Watchers oatmeal packets are a decent alternative)

- High-fiber, low-sugar breakfast cereal (Kashi and All-Bran, as noted earlier, are good choices) with milk

Accessories
- 2 links turkey sausage
- 2 slices ham
- 3 slices bacon
- 4 ounces lean ground beef
- Whole-wheat toast or bagel
- Yogurt with less than 15 grams of sugar per serving

Fruits
- Apple
- Banana
- Orange
- Kiwi
- Peach
- Handful of berries (blue-, straw-, black-, or rasp-)

I encourage you to spice up your food. Bland food makes you feel bad about yourself. Feel free to add pepper and/or a dash of salt to your eggs. Hot sauce is fine. Try some cinnamon, nutmeg, or allspice in your oatmeal, or add a packet of Splenda if it's not sweet enough for you. If you're using a vanilla protein supplement you like a lot, you can add a scoop to your oatmeal or to plain yogurt.

On the days when you don't even have the aforementioned five to seven minutes to get ready, try this "Oh, crap, I'm late!" shake:

2 scoops vanilla protein powder
½ cup rolled oats
1 cup berries

1 teaspoon Splenda

½-1 cup water (depending on how thick you like your shakes)

Blend it, pour it in a cup, and drink it on the way to work.

IMMEDIATELY AFTER YOUR WORKOUT

You can buy supplemental protein powder two different ways. Some formulas contain flavored protein and nothing else, while others are "meal replacement" supplements. The latter contain carbs and sometimes fat along with the protein. They're generally more expensive, but they make postworkout nutrition relatively simple: just add water and shake, and you have all you need.

If you're using protein alone, you still shake it up with water. But you should add a carbohydrate source. It doesn't have to be complicated; a banana or handful of raisins will work.

You can also get fancier and throw either type of supplement into a blender with water and fresh or frozen fruit. That adds extra calories, but also makes your postworkout shake into more of a treat.

I can't tell you which protein formulations are the best, except to note that the cheapest ones probably won't taste very good, and may not work particularly well for you. The good ones cost more, mainly because high-quality ingredients are really expensive.

I recommend experimenting with a few, buying them in the smallest possible quantities until you figure out which one suits you best. (Gastrointestinal disturbance is a pretty good sign that the offending supplement isn't right for you.) My favorite postworkout mix is Surge from Biotest, which can be found at biotest.net.

For some of you, protein supplements are out of the question. Some people won't touch them on principle. (I'm not sure which principle it is, exactly, but I've met people who're adamant about not using supplements.) Others just can't afford them. I've been broke, so I can relate.

The smart play for nonsupplementers is to get some protein of any type ASAP following a workout. For example, two eight-ounce cartons of milk from a convenience store will give you 16 grams of protein, including branched-chain amino acids, the protein components most directly associated with building muscle. Another good choice, if you can enjoy it without gagging, is cottage cheese, which I mentioned earlier in this chapter. Also, if you're working out at home, consider some postworkout scrambled eggs and toast. It doesn't matter if you've already had breakfast; eggs are a great protein source any time of day.

And if none of those is a realistic option, grab anything that has protein and carbs, even if it's just a hamburger.

LUNCH AND DINNER

I can't possibly guess what you like or can afford to eat, or what you're willing to do to prepare the things you like to eat. So I'll keep this simple: for lunch and dinner, you want to pick one thing from each of these categories:

- major protein source (beef, pork, chicken, turkey, fish);
- significant volume of vegetables (at least one cup of raw or cooked vegetables, or a salad) or a piece of fruit;
- one other carb source (whole-grain bread, potato, rice, pasta).

You may note that I included potatoes here with the bread and pasta, whereas I listed them with vegetables earlier. That's because potatoes are a relatively dense source of carbohydrate calories, meaning they're more like bread than broccoli.

Sandwiches are part of our lives, and they just happen to fit this model, within reason. A ham-and-Swiss sandwich with lettuce and tomatoes on whole-wheat bread covers the bases. Sure, in a perfect world more vegetables and less bread would be better, but I don't live in that world, and you probably don't either.

If you like to cook, or are simply willing to cook yourself a decent meal every now and then, I recommend making enough food for two, three, or four meals, and having the leftovers for lunch or dinner later in the week (for tasty, easy-to-prepare, guy-friendly recipes, check out builtforshow.com).

I'll leave the volume of food up to you. Just eat more when you're trying to pack on muscle, and cut back on carbs and excess fats (like mayonnaise and salad dressings) when you're trying to get lean for summer. I don't believe in overeating or starving yourself to make big changes in your body weight in a short amount of time. If you can gain four or five pounds of muscle a month when you're bulking up, and lose a pound or two of fat a week when you're trying to cut, you'll get noticeable results without extreme fluctuations that might screw up your metabolism in the long run.

SNACKS

We need something to tide us over between lunch and dinner. Here are a few snacks that are simple and easy to tote around and eat at work or in your car:

- two pieces of string cheese with some baby carrots;
- one or two handfuls of almonds or cashews, skim milk, and a piece of fruit;
- a protein or meal-replacement bar with a piece of fruit;

In the last category, I recommend Bumble or Lara bars, which you can find in the health-food section of your grocery store. I also like Metabolic Drive Cookie Dough bars from Biotest.

Part 4. When to eat, specifically

Ideally, you'll eat a meal or snack every three to four hours; you'll keep your metabolism ramped up and your hunger pangs ratcheted down. If you feel ravenously hungry at any point, you've waited too long.

Here's what a meal schedule might look like on a perfect day. Obviously, that schedule will change depending on when you work out, so I wrote it two different ways.

WITH MORNING WORKOUT:

WAKE UP: 7 a.m.

BREAKFAST: 7:30 a.m.

WORKOUT: 8:30–9:30 a.m.

POSTWORKOUT SHAKE: 9:30 a.m., or within thirty minutes of finishing

LUNCH: between noon and 1 p.m.

SNACK: between 3 and 4 p.m.

DINNER: between 6 and 7:30 p.m.

WITH EVENING WORKOUT:

WAKE UP: 7 a.m.

BREAKFAST: 7:30 a.m.

SNACK: between 10 and 11 a.m.

LUNCH: between 1 and 2 p.m.

WORKOUT: 5–6 p.m.

POSTWORKOUT SHAKE: 6 p.m., or within thirty minutes of finishing

DINNER: between 7 and 8 p.m.

How do you manage all those meals and snacks if you're away from home all day? I recommend a small plastic cooler that you can keep in your car and/or tote into the office, or one of those flexible cooler pouches that you can carry in your backpack or gym bag. The former isn't subtle, and might raise eyebrows if you work in an office with lots of people who couldn't spell "nutrition" if you spotted them two *n*'s, two *t*'s, and two *i*'s. But if they ask about it, you can always tell them the truth: you keep a spare kidney in the cooler. Bonus points if you wink and add, "You never know when the boss might need one."

Part 5. Final words, about alcohol

In Chapter 3, I proposed a weekly limit of five drinks and said you can choose how and when to drink them—a drink with dinner five nights a week, or all five on a Saturday night.

A few more specifics:

- Stay away from fruity drinks. They're loaded with sugar, and might have more than 300 calories per drink.

- If you're drinking hard liquor, be a man and drink it straight. If you have to mix it, use club soda or a diet soft drink.
- White wine is okay, but red has slightly less sugar, and might be better for you overall.
- If beer is your beverage of choice, make it light beer.
- Never, under any circumstance, order a Cosmopolitan. That's more of a personal rule, though.

CHAPTER TEN

How to Flaunt What You Have and Hide What You Don't

I am not by any stretch of the imagination an authority on men's fashion; I leave that complicated stuff to the guys at *GQ,* master pickup artists, and, on certain family occasions, my mother.

But since I pick my own clothes (with a lot of help from some very patient girlfriends), and haven't been laughed out of the clubs just yet, I figure I know enough to get in the game. And that's fine by me.

If you can remember all the way back to Chapter 3, I wrote about the mindset that keeps skinny guys skinny and fat guys fat. In this chapter, I tell you about the ways skinny guys present themselves that make them look even skinnier, and how fat guys don't do themselves any favors by wearing clothes that call attention to the most unappealing aspects of their shape.

First, though, I want to give equal time to guys who're built exactly the way most of us want to be built—lean and muscular—but dress themselves in clothes so tight you suspect they shop at the boys' department of Old Navy. And then there's that scowl we've all seen, the one that says, "I can bench-press your mom's minivan," or "I'm in the middle of taking a dump the size of a Caribbean archipelago." Either way, it's a look that says to women, "I'd rather intimidate total strangers than get intimate with you."

Bottom line, all of us could do better in the self-presentation department.

FIRST, A FEW TIPS THAT APPLY TO EVERYONE

DON'T BREAK THE MOST BASIC RULES OF FASHION AND STYLE

Your mother probably told you that your shoes and belt should match. It may be the oldest and most inviolable tenet of male fashion. Here are some others that may not be quite so obvious or so often repeated:

- A shirt or jacket sleeve should never extend past the base of your thumb. And it should always reach your wrist joint. That leaves you with maybe an inch of wiggle room in between those two points. If for financial reasons you have to wear the shirts you have, and some of those shirts are too long, keep the sleeves rolled up to disguise the misfit.

- Socks and shoes should achieve some sort of harmony. Don't wear athletic socks with dress shoes, or vice versa, unless you're trying to collect disability insurance because of that box that fell on your head in the company warehouse. In that case, feel free to take your fashion cues from the cast of *The Ringer*.

- Your socks shouldn't show when you're standing up. Too-short pants have a magical ability to make skinny guys look skinnier (picture Pee-wee Herman if you don't believe me), fat guys look fatter, and short guys look shorter. Even well-built guys who're taller than average will look like country bumpkins with pants that stop short of the tops of their shoes. It's like you're still wearing your wardrobe from before you hit your last growth spurt. That's okay when you're twelve. It's creepy when you're twenty-four.

- Pants that are too long aren't as much of an issue. If they drag on the floor, yeah, that looks stupid, but an extra inch on the bottom isn't something that's going to set off a woman's dork-o-meter. As in so many other things in life, it's better to be an inch too long than an inch too short.

- Here's a fashion rule I didn't know until I stumbled across it while doing research for this chapter: technically, your socks are supposed to match your trousers, rather than your shoes. But this may be the fashion rule most often violated by non-dorky men. Look around, and you'll probably see lots of otherwise well-dressed guys who ignore it. So I'm back to what I said earlier about trouser length: the less people see of your socks, the better. But whatever they see should at least match one thing or another—your pants or your shoes. (And do I even need to add that socks should also match each other?)

HATS ARE FOR BALL GAMES

Baseball caps are okay as long as they're clean, not backward, and not combined with anything you might wear to a job interview. Regardless of the fashion trend of the moment, wearing your cap off-center, especially if the bill of the cap is flat instead of curved, lowers your presumed IQ by at least one standard deviation.

And trust me on this one: you can't get away with a fedora or cowboy hat just because you saw your favorite rock star doing it. He looks cool in it. You don't.

LOGOS ARE FOR NASCAR

Don't cover yourself head to toe in logos. It makes you look like you never left high school. If you're wearing a baseball cap with a school or team or company logo on it, try not to wear anything else that reflects a public or private entity's branding strategy. You're trying to create your own brand, not link yourself to someone else's.

WHITE ISN'T ALWAYS RIGHT

When guys like us look in the mirror, as often as not it's to make sure there aren't any new zits that need to be zapped. That's why we aren't as observant as we should be when it comes to our shirts. We might miss a fleck of pasta sauce on our favorite white shirt, and then compound the problem by washing and drying the shirt without taking steps to get the damned spot out. The ironic result of washing a shirt with a tiny spot is that we ensure that the spot doesn't ever come out. It's "set," as my mom would say, and it'll be there as long as you own that shirt.

So what's the problem? Shit happens, right? Yes, shit does happen, but when it happens in tiny increments, you may not notice it. Women will. No woman would mark a guy down for getting a spot on his shirt, but if she sees him more than once with the same spot on the same shirt, she'll most definitely deduct points from the score sheet. And if you're a borderline player in her book, she'll bounce you back to the minor leagues without your even realizing that you've been up to bat.

The lesson: Don't wear anything white unless you're 100 percent confident in your laundry skills.

CHECKS AREN'T REALLY FLATTERING ON ANYBODY

They make skinny guys look weak and fat guys look like they've given up. Even if you're buff, they hide your muscles. It's the fashion equivalent of a potato sack.

LEAN, WELL-BUILT GUYS CAN GET AWAY WITH CONTRASTING COLORS

A white shirt with black pants (as long as you aren't having pasta for dinner), a red shirt with jeans, navy blue with khakis . . . As long as you aren't mixing patterns (vertical and horizontal stripes, say), a guy with an athletic build has a lot more leeway than a guy whose physique is still a work in progress.

But enough about guys like that. Let's look at some strategies for guys who're in the process of transforming themselves but aren't quite there yet.

FOR SKINNY GUYS WHO ARE PUTTING ON MUSCLE

A TIGHTER T-SHIRT MAKES A SKINNY GUY LOOK BIGGER

Just don't get "tighter" confused with "small." You should never look like you're wearing someone else's clothes. A T-shirt should be formfitting, but not skintight.

Length matters. You want a T-shirt to hang just past your belt line, but no farther. The ones that go down below your crotch make it look like you're trying to hide an unfortunate stain in the middle of your pelvic region. And if they go even lower than that, you start to look like a middle-school girl at a sleepover.

SWEATERS GIVE YOUR UPPER TORSO MORE SHAPE THAN IT ACTUALLY HAS

In our grandparents' generation, the sight of a well-endowed young woman in a sweater was as close as they got to Internet porn. This is a lesson guys can use: a sweater makes your chest look bigger, your shoulders look wider, and your arms look thicker. Layers in general enhance a thin frame. Obviously, this tip is seasonal and situational. You can't wear your favorite sweater to a barbecue in July no matter how good it makes your shoulders look.

NEVER WEAR A SHIRT OR JACKET THAT DOESN'T FIT YOUR SHOULDERS SQUARELY

The worst for skinny guys is when the stitching that attaches the sleeve to the rest of the shirt hangs halfway down your deltoids. Even if you're lean and in good shape (not skinny-fat, in other words), a shirt that's too big for your shoulders makes you look like you raided your big brother's closet. Or, worse, that you just emerged from the hospital after barely surviving a near-fatal disease. Nobody would guess that you picked that shirt for yourself, and no woman wants to be seen with a guy who doesn't dress himself.

Wearing a shirt or jacket that's too small in the shoulders doesn't do you any favors either. Once again, I ask you to think of Pee-wee Herman, and remember to do the opposite.

Your only choice is to pick shirts, jackets, and sweaters with a shoulder seam that actually fits your shoulders. You want it to go right to the edge of your shoulders, but no farther.

Whether or not to wear a T-shirt underneath a dress shirt or sweater is a judgment call. However, if you have protruding collarbones, I think an undershirt is pretty much required.

TROUSERS SHOULD WORK WITH THE ILLUSION CREATED BY YOUR SHIRT AND/OR SWEATER

One of the benefits of being skinny is that you can wear tighter jeans, like the classic Levi's 501s. (They're the ones with the red tag.) Levi's are to buttocks what sweaters are to pecs. If you don't believe me, ask a hot-looking woman. You may not spend a minute of your life thinking about what your butt looks like in jeans, but women do.

So when the weather's warm, combine formfitting jeans with a formfitting T-shirt and you may find that you're already more built for show than you ever imagined. Conversely, a tight T-shirt combined with baggy jeans or shorts ruins the effect. Just remember that, as with your T-shirt, there is such a thing as "too tight." Leave something to the imagination.

When the weather's cold and you're using a shirt and sweater to thicken your upper body, you need to switch to relaxed-fit jeans or khakis to continue the illusion. The worst combination is tight, straight-legged jeans on the lower half, with seven layers (topped by a down vest) on the upper half. I don't know if anyone south, east, or west of Montana dresses this way, but just in case they do, I want to advise them otherwise, as a public service.

LIGHTER COLORS MAKE YOU LOOK MORE BUFF

Light blues and greens, for whatever reasons, work best for skinny guys. I advise against tangerine and pink, unless you're really brave or travel in the kind of company where choices like that are accepted.

On the negative side, black makes you look even skinnier than you are. Unless you're auditioning for a Ramones tribute band, forget the black T-shirt and black jeans.

DITCH THE WALLET

If you're skinny, you want women to look in the general direction of your back pockets. And you don't want anything, least of all the rectangular lump of your wallet, distorting and spoiling the view.

Look, you don't even need to carry a wallet when you're out on the town. All you need is an ID, a credit card, and cash, all of which you can carry together in a front pocket, with or without a money clip.

BIG SHOES MAKE EVERYTHING ELSE LOOK SMALLER

Wide, chunky shoes are a terrible idea—they emphasize everything about you that isn't big or chunky. Anything bigger than Skechers is almost certainly a mistake.

FOR HEAVIER GUYS WHO ARE GETTING LEANER

EXPLORE THE DARK SIDE

Since light colors make thin guys look more muscular and athletic, you can figure that dark colors have a similar effect for guys carrying more weight than they want. A black button-down shirt could have made Henry VIII look like a NutriSystem success story.

WHATEVER YOU WEAR, IT MUST FIT PERFECTLY

Loose clothing makes you look even bigger than you are, while tight clothes give away curves that you don't want exposed.

CHOOSE YOUR PATTERNS WISELY

Checks make you look fatter. Horizontal stripes make you look fatter *and* shorter. Vertical stripes can have the opposite effect. If you pick a shirt with subtle vertical stripes, or a pin-striped suit if you need to wear such a thing, you can make your body look longer and leaner.

But it only works if it's subtle. Taking fashion risks with colors and patterns almost always ends up emphasizing your girth, for reasons I can't really explain. It's just the way it is. Boring clothes that fit well are much more flattering than interesting clothes.

LAYERS AREN'T IN YOUR BEST INTEREST

In winter, pick one comfortable and flattering long-sleeved shirt, preferably black or at least dark. That's your club shirt. It doesn't have to be button-down; a pullover can work as well, as long as it's not overly tight around your midsection. (If the shirt moves when your belly jiggles, it's too tight.)

A lot of big guys I've known won't step outside their apartment without wearing an undershirt. I understand if you have a demonstrable perspiration problem and need something to soak it up. But if it's just a habit, or if you're wearing the undershirt as a psychological shield against people seeing your actual dimensions, I recommend a new strategy. The less covering you put over your girth, the less girth you'll appear to have.

LOSE YOUR BAGGAGE

I mentioned earlier that skinny guys should never carry a thick wallet in a back pocket. For big guys, the rule applies to every pocket. If you stop to think about it, there's hardly anything you really need to carry around in pockets. Cash, credit card, ID in one front pocket. Cell phone in the other front pocket. A pen and your car key in whichever front pocket works best. (BTW, unless you're a janitor, why would you need to carry more than one or two keys with you everywhere you go? If you need multiple house keys, carry them in your briefcase or backpack at work, and lock them in your car when you're out with your friends.) Add a handkerchief to one of your back pockets, and that's all you need. Anything else just creates bulges that call attention to the bigger bulge hanging over your belt.

FINALLY, A FEW WORDS ABOUT CONFIDENCE

I hope this is obvious, but I'll say it anyway, just in case it isn't: my object in this chapter isn't to make you feel bad about your body, your clothes, or your personal sense of style (assuming you have one). I also didn't do it for the sake of enriching the garment industry. I know what it's like to have maxed-out credit cards, and the last thing I want is to make you think you have to start pumping plastic until you've upgraded your wardrobe from top to bottom.

We're all in transition here. The best we can do is work with what we have. And chances are, you already have more than you realize. I've talked to more women than I can remember, and I'm proud to say, I'm not too bad in the chatting-up-strangers department. I didn't have to wait until I was built for show, or until I had managed to accumulate a closet filled with clothes my mother hadn't picked out for me. You don't either. The key to all this is to carry yourself with confidence.

Confidence can't be faked, but it can be built up over time, just like strength and muscle mass. We've all known guys who were pure bluster, with phony confidence bordering on cockiness. You knew they were faking it, and you can bet the women they tried to impress know they were faking it as well.

So how do you start building confidence? First, as I've hinted throughout this chapter, you want to focus more on what you have and less on what you don't have (yet). In a way, it's the opposite of dressing for success: don't dress like a buff guy if you aren't. But at the same time, you do yourself a favor if you play up your best qualities, the things you like about yourself, while consciously keeping the focus off the things you're working to improve. You can dislike being skinny or fat without disliking yourself for being either of those things.

Take it from me: no matter how hard you train, and no matter how carefully you monitor your diet, there'll probably never be a day when you look in the mirror and say to yourself, "Damn! I'm totally perfect!" You'll always see something in the mirror you want to work on, and that's the way it should be. Research has shown that the best athletes in the world keep working on the skills they haven't yet mastered to their own satisfaction, while the also-rans spend much more time in their comfort zone, practicing the things they're already good at doing. If you're serious about self-improvement, you'll continue to work on the parts of yourself that are the most problematic.

You're already taking steps to address your weaknesses, and you should congratulate yourself for that. Just keep in mind, as I said earlier, that you still have to play the game, even while your physique is in transition. The way you do it is to acknowledge that you're a fine and interesting person even without the body you want, or clothes that work perfectly with the body you have. You have to like yourself now, without falling into the trap of thinking that you'll like yourself better when you take two more inches off your waist or add a few centimeters to your upper arms.

Women are more attracted to confident guys than they are to guys who radiate insecurity, either by shrinking away or by overcompensating with bombast. You don't have to call attention to your weaknesses. Just do yourself a favor and keep the focus on your strengths. Women will like you more if they get the sense that you like yourself.

None of this negates the message of *Built for Show*. Experience and science agree on this point: a leaner, more muscular, more powerful-looking physique makes you more attractive to women. When I talk about the importance of confidence, I'm talking about another aspect of the process. There's a difference between what catches a woman's eye and what engages her heart and mind.

Yeah, all else being equal, the guy with the better body is going to get more chances to step up to the plate, and the umpires in life will give him more chances to score. To continue the baseball analogy past its expiration date, a skinny or fat guy might be called out on the first strike, whereas the guy with the great physique gets all the way to "strike five" before he's sent to the showers. That part of life isn't fair. Never has been, never will be.

But without confidence, you may not have any better luck with five strikes than you did with one. Alwyn Cosgrove, a friend of mine in the training business, tells the story of a client who lost one hundred pounds of fat. His profile literally went from fat to flat; the dude had ripped abs and everything. But the guy still had so little confidence in himself that he refused to take off his shirt in public, and had the farmer's tan lines to prove it.

It's not just the guys who've made transformations who become disconnected from the reality of their appearance. I have friends who are funny, smart, good-looking, and on their way to successful careers who seem to shrink away if they're around a beautiful woman.

You don't have to be either of those guys.

To my way of thinking, the key is to start building confidence now, rather than waiting. If you know you're only going to get one chance, you'd better make the most of it. The better you do with your limited opportunities now, the more you'll enjoy your expanded opportunities later.

To put it another way, the more you like yourself now, the more fun you'll have then.

CHAPTER ELEVEN

Presenting . . . You!

omen everywhere are trying to tell you something important: They want you.

Most of us just aren't listening.

We like to think we're the ones on the prowl, that we fire the first shot and give women the chance to return fire. But women are much better at this game than we are. They have dozens of ways to encourage one of us to take a shot, which means they're making observations about us before we've noticed them. Simply, they've had more practice.

This chapter focuses on meeting and attracting women while displaying your best qualities. As was the case in Chapter 10, when I shared my limited expertise in fashion, I'm not trying to pass myself off as an expert on picking up women. (If you want real experts' advice on that subject, see the relevant titles listed in "Resources and Recommended Reading," beginning on page 233.) But I have done some reading and fieldwork in this area, and from time to time I've brought my work home with me, including a professional model, an adult-film actress, and more than my share of women who don't make a living with their looks but could.

As I said back in Chapter 4, a lot of things are out of your control once you step into Hookup World. You're being judged on your facial symmetry and height—two dynamics that were mostly decided at conception, nine months before you even crapped your first diaper—as well as your perceived wealth, education level, and social status.

But even if you, like me, lack height (I'm five feet nine), wealth, education (the only degree I have is an antiperspirant), and other markers of social status, you can get by on the two aces we all keep in our deck: our physiques, and our personalities. Just about everything else in *BFS* has been about improving your physique, for good reason. And I don't want to say that "personality" is something you can or should strive to change in any substantial way. As with your height and facial symmetry, you are who your parents' sperm and egg decided you would be. But all of us can project a more positive, likable, and attractive version of that personality to the outside world. Which, as you guessed, is the subject of this chapter.

PREP WORK

MASTER YOURSELF

Neil Strauss, author of the bestselling pickup memoir *The Game,* was a skinny, balding, awkward man who talked way too fast and couldn't get a single date. Now he's hailed as one of the greatest pickup artists in the world. While changing his physical appearance helped him make the transition from geek to sleek, it was the concept he called "inner game" that was the crucial turning point. You can sum it up like this: before you can approach a quality woman, you have to feel like a quality man.

If that seems beyond your reach right now, go back and review the "Confidence" section of Chapter 10. It may even help to write down a list of your best qualities and the best events of your life so far. Keep the list in a place where you'll see it regularly. Refer to it often, and add to it when you feel inspired.

HAVE STANDARDS

Some guys will sleep with any woman who shows interest. I'm sure it saves time and money, but it also lowers your self-image, and the way others perceive you. Others will start off an evening chatting up and getting shot down by the top-shelf babes. Then they'll work their way down the evolutionary scale until they find someone as desperate as they are. That approach doesn't save time or money—if anything, it takes longer and costs more—and the result may be even worse for your confidence and for the desperation you project to your peers.

You will not be either of those guys.

Here's another assignment for you: Write a short paragraph about who your ideal date is. Not who it is you'd settle for after ten shots of Jägermeister, and not the Hooters waitress you thought about when you masturbated into a banana peel last night. Who would you want to hang out with? What does she look like? What kind of qualities does she have? Is she athletic? Funny? Close to her family? Is she a local woman, or someone who's new in town? How much education does she have? Be as specific as possible about the qualities you find attractive in a woman you're likely to encounter.

Below that paragraph, write down three deal breakers. Could you never see yourself with someone who smokes, or drinks you under the table, or has a habit that requires 2 a.m. trips to the local trailer park? Are you turned off by someone who hates exercise? Do you find certain personality traits or personal habits annoying?

But don't write down more than three turnoffs. You aren't perfect, and there's no such thing as a perfect woman seeking a meaningful relationship with an imperfect guy. Courtships and relationships are always about give-and-take, and you don't want to put up too many roadblocks.

The most important part of this exercise is to figure out what you want, and remind yourself what you could never settle for. Why is that important? Because most of what follows assumes that you're looking to make the best possible first impression, and keep open the chance of that first impression leading to some first-night carnality. I just want you to keep in mind that you have standards, and your standards for a one-night stand shouldn't be lower than your ideal for a long-term relationship. It's unlikely that a successful hookup will lead to that kind of ongoing romance, but it might. And it's completely possible that a first meeting *not* resulting in a hookup could lead to an exchange of phone numbers, dates, and an actual relationship.

In either event, it's crucial that your standards start high and stay high.

CHECK YOUR POSTURE

Poor posture can negate the dynamic, athletic look you've been developing with the *BFS* workouts. It suggests a lack of confidence, and accentuates all the parts of your body you'd rather not accentuate. To assess your posture, stand with your back to a wall, making sure your head, shoulders, butt, and heels all touch the wall, but not the backs of your knees.

Does this feel natural? Can you stand like this for a few minutes? Can you turn your head from left to right, as you would in a conversation? Can you cross your arms in front of your chest, or put your fingers in your front pockets, as you would in a conversation, and still keep your head, shoulders, butt, and heels in contact with the wall?

If not, try this: squeeze your shoulder blades together, like you're trying to pinch something between them, and drop them like you're putting them in your back pockets. Make sure your head remains level. Now put one hand behind the small of your back. If you can fit your whole hand between your back and the wall—especially if it fits without actually touching your back or the wall—you know you created a new problem (too much curve in your lower back, which pushes your belly out) to fix another (shoulders slumping forward).

To fix it, squeeze your abs and bring your belly back in. That should close the gap between your lower back and the wall. Stand like that, breathing deeply and steadily, for a minute or two. For some guys, simply standing up straight and breathing will feel like an ab workout. That's a sign that the deepest muscles of your abdominal wall are weaker than they should be, and it's affecting your posture—which in turn affects the first impression you give the women you meet.

Step away from the wall, maintaining that same posture. See if you can keep your shoulders back and your midsection tight while walking around your living room. If it doesn't feel natural—if you suspect that you look like a guy sitting on a fence post—repeat the wall drill every day, or even multiple times a day, until you can stand tall without thinking about it.

BEFORE YOU GO OUT

GET YOUR PUMP ON

Ever notice how good you look and feel after you just finish a workout? Of course you do! Your muscles are full of blood, you have energy to burn, and you probably feel borderline euphoric. It's your instant reward for training, and it's what makes you look forward to the next workout.

You can replicate that sensation with the following "pregame" routine. It should take you two minutes, at most, and it's best to do it right before you jump into the shower. That leaves you primed for a night on the town.

1. Do ten body-weight squats with your hands behind your head.
2. Immediately do five to ten push-ups.
3. Repeat four more times, with no rest in between exercises.
4. Hit the shower.

GET YOUR HEAD IN THE GAME

When you're done washing up, put on some good, upbeat music and get dressed in your favorite outfit. Dab on a little cologne. Check your nostrils for any rogue hairs and your teeth for any stray food particles. Now would be a good time to read over your list of your best qualities. Close your eyes, smile, and imagine how much fun you're going to have meeting people and hanging with friends. Clap your hands together. It's game time.

AT THE SCENE

You're at the club. You've met your friends. (Or you're flying solo.) What next?

MAKE IT CLEAR THAT YOU'RE AVAILABLE

- If you're trying to look cool, don't. This is the time to look friendly and inviting. Show some teeth; guys who don't smile don't get the girl.

- When you're moving, don't prowl around the venue like Elmer Fudd stalking Bugs Bunny. It lowers your perceived social value, and every woman in the club now knows exactly what you're after. If you're with friends, get a conversation going. If you move from one spot to another, try to engage someone in a friendly chat, even if it's just another group of guys or some couples with no hookup potential. It doesn't matter what you talk about, or for how long. The main reason is to get in the mood to talk, giving you some momentum for the conversations you'll soon have—the ones that really do offer hookup potential. The secondary reason is to signal that you're a popular, magnetic guy, even if you didn't actually know a single person in the room before you walked into it. (If you want to do some pregame research, check out *The Wedding Crashers*. Yeah, it's a comedy, but you might take away some tips for chatting up strangers.)

- When you're sitting, don't land in a spot where it's hard for females to approach you. Unless you're a celebrity, no woman is going to maneuver through a crowd to see if there's any mutual interest. So instead of angling for a corner, find a spot in an open area. Once you're there, lean back, look relaxed, and take up some space. Spread out a little. Laugh at your buddies' jokes. Make it clear that you're having fun, and that there's room for someone to join you.

- When you see a woman you're interested in, make eye contact. If she returns it, it's time for the next phase.

CATCH THE SIGNS THAT SHE'S INTERESTED

This whole process would be sweet and easy if women just told us what was up: "Hi, you look interesting. Let's have a drink so I can figure out if you're okay or if you remind me of my last boyfriend, who turned out to be a total dick."

Alas, it's all based on subtle signs and cues—signals that most of us miss if we don't know what to look for, or misinterpret what we see. To make it more difficult for both of you, she may not even realize she's tipping her hand. A few common signs, aside from basic eye contact:

- gazing in your direction more than once;
- making eye contact and smiling;
- licking her lips;
- tossing her hair;
- establishing a closer physical proximity.

Now, don't get too excited and think that every woman who does one of the aforementioned is showing interest. Sometimes she tosses her hair because it's in her eyes. Sometimes she moves closer because there's nowhere else to stand. Sometimes the eye contact and smile are directed at the guy standing behind you. But if you see a combination of these signs, or one particularly noticeable cue that she repeats, chances are good that she's open to you approaching her. The signs don't mean anything more than that—not yet, anyway. But they do give you a chance.

MAKE YOUR FIRST MOVE

The longer you wait to make contact, the more importance you give it. A mostly random and probably fruitless encounter assumes more emotional weight than any reasonable person would assign to it. With importance comes anxiety, and with anxiety comes inaction . . . followed by more anxiety, followed by regret when another guy catches her attention and moves in.

That's why Mystery, a pickup artist and author of *The Mystery Method,* recommends "the three-second rule." When someone offers a sign of interest, simply approach her. If several women in a group look your way, make immediate contact. In her eyes, or their collective eyes, you're friendly and confident. In your own mind, you've bypassed the instinct to psyche yourself up for a move, since you haven't given that thought a chance to form.

So what do you say when you approach her? Let's start with what *not* to say: pickup lines are really just comedic one-liners that have never *and will never* work. Besides, if the woman you're trying to talk with is attractive enough to catch your attention, she's already heard a million of them. You can't pique her interest unless you offer something the other guys she's shot down already didn't have.

Your worst play is to compliment her looks. She's not confused about the effect she has on men; she's probably dressed and accessorized and made herself up to accentuate her most attractive qualities . . . which, of course, is exactly what I told you to do in the previous chapter. So you're both working from the same playbook. Besides—and this is absolutely essential to understand—complimenting her looks is giving her credit for something that was largely out of her control. It also suggests that your attraction to her is largely out of your control. You're saying, in effect, "I find you biologically suitable to bear my children"—without giving her any reason to consider you for the job of fathering those children. It's the conversational equivalent of grinding your crotch into her backside the first time you hit the dance floor.

Your second-worst play is to be the survey taker, the one who asks boring questions ("What's your name?" "Come here often?") that she's been asked and has answered more times than she could remember.

There's no single conversational gambit that's going to work every time, which is why it's so important to jump right in before you've had time to think of one. Try an offhanded comment about something your friend and you were just talking about. If you get the sense that she's into music, tell her you've been thinking about a particular song all day, but can't remember what it is or who sings it. If she looks like a sports fan, draw her into a conversation about one of the local teams.

Remember, the purpose of an opening comment is to generate rapport and start an open-ended conversation.

GET A CONVERSATION STARTED

If you were out in the wilderness and your very survival depended on starting a fire and keeping it going, you'd build that fire slowly and carefully. You'd start with tinder, add some twigs, and gradually work your way up to bigger and thicker chunks of wood that burn hotter and longer.

Your approach to the conversation should work the same way. Your opening comment put flame on the tinder, and now you need to feed it with twigs until you have a steady blaze going. Body language is crucial here. Facing her directly and crowding into her personal space is too aggressive, like dumping logs onto tinder. Besides, you don't know yet if she's the right person to squeeze into *your* personal space. Remember, you have standards, and all you know about her right now is that there's a flicker of attraction.

Here you want to talk over your shoulder, while making eye-to-eye contact when you speak. This part of the conversation is the equivalent of feeding twigs to the tinder, and letting the flame build. After a couple of minutes, when it's clear she doesn't want you to leave, and you're pretty sure you don't want her to leave, feel free to face her more directly and give her more of your attention.

KEEP THE CONVERSATION GOING

Tonality is huge in a conversation. Do you talk so fast that even your friends have trouble keeping up? Slow it down. Can you tell she's having trouble understanding you? Use fewer words. And, um, while we're on the subject of, you know, um, kind of annoying conversational—oh, what the hell's the word I'm looking for here?—tics! That's it! Are you one of those guys who puts two or three completely unnecessary fillers like "like" or, you know, "you know" into every sentence, no matter how short or simple the idea you're trying to express? Are you a guy with a lot of verbal tics, like the need to say "um um um" or "and, uh" whenever you're trying to make a transition from one thought to the next? All these fillers and tics insert themselves into our conversations without us noticing, but a complete stranger will notice them, and probably find them annoying.

An even worse habit is to carry on a conversation with yourself in the middle of a conversation with someone you've just met. Asking yourself questions ("What's the word I'm looking for here?"), chuckling at your own clever word-play (really, it's probably not that clever), or any other indication that you don't really need a second person to have a dialogue is a pretty good way to ensure that you'll have no shortage of opportunities to talk to yourself.

All these conversation-stoppers are signs that you're more focused on what you're trying to say than on how she's responding to what you're saying. I don't mean that in a mean way. Each of us has the potential to turn into a babbling nitwit when we're trying to impress someone we've just met.

You can debug your conversational habits with some practice, including the practice you get from chatting up lots of people in lots of situations. But you can also take the tension out of conversations by remembering a simple fact about this type of conversation: what you say isn't nearly as important as how you say it. Your posture, your eye contact, and the confidence you project are all a lot more important than the wit or profundity of your words. So, really, the pressure's off; there's no need to babble or fill the air with sounds or search for specific words. Focus on her instead of on you, and you'll come off much better.

STEADILY INCREASE EYE CONTACT

Eye contact is crucial. An inability to keep your eyes focused on her face during a first conversation means you're not going to get a chance to focus your eyes on any other part of her. But staring too hard eye-to-eye is creepy. So it's okay to look at her mouth when she's speaking, and it's okay to glance away briefly during a shift in the conversation as you're collecting a thought. But when you're speaking to her, you must make eye contact. If you're constantly looking around the room she'll get the message that you're nervous, or that you'd rather be somewhere else.

Speaking of eye contact, if you wear glasses, make sure they're clean. Women like to be able to see a man's eyes. Here's a trick: If you're chatting up a woman who appears interested, take off your glasses and casually wipe off the lenses while maintaining eye contact with her. That gives her a preview of what your eyes will look like in bed, when you won't be wearing your glasses.

SHORTEN THE DISTANCE BETWEEN YOU

Leaning forward during a conversation is a way to foreshadow intimacy. But there are good and bad ways to do this. Cocking your head forward without moving anything else makes you look like a bird, and if done too early in the interaction comes off as needy. Leaning your shoulders in is the better play.

I don't want to make you too focused on your posture, because if you do you'll probably end up looking unnatural and uncomfortable. And when you're at this stage of the process, "uncomfortable" is the last quality you want to convey. So when I advise you to lean your shoulders in, I don't suggest doing so at the expense of your posture by rounding your upper back. It's better to lean from the waist or hips, so you keep your posture while also getting your shoulders in closer to the object of your interest.

Another way to use your body language to signal interest—and I'd never have guessed this if I hadn't heard it from someone who swears he learned it in a sociology class—is to show the inside of your wrists. It's a sign of friendly intentions in all cultures. Since I heard that, I've observed how people talk to each other when no one's trying to establish dominance. You'll see people turn their palms up during conversations, a gesture that inadvertently exposes the inside of the wrists. But when arguing or scolding, people tend to make sharper, harder, finger-pointing gestures, which show the back of the forearm, rather than the nicer, lighter, less hairy side. So, while this tip won't make or break a potentially intimate encounter, it never hurts to throw in a gesture of friendly intent.

MAKE INCIDENTAL CONTACT

Incidental contact is a crucial step in the dance. Briefly, casually, and lightly (*lightly!*) touching her arm during a conversation can advertise your interest in going further without being too aggressive. It also puts the ball in her court. If she returns incidental contact, you're moving forward. (If she screams for the bouncer, walk away. Quickly.)

SYNCOPATE YOUR DRINKING STYLES

Try to show as much interest in and fondness for alcohol as she does. She doesn't have to match you drink for drink, but you should at least keep up with her. That said, if she puts three down while you're still working on your first, you're clearly dealing with a serious drinker here, and there's no pressure to keep up if you're out of your depth. A hard-drinking woman isn't necessarily an alcoholic—she could just be a Russian tennis player—but whatever chance you have will be lost if she discovers that she can drink you under the table.

The key to matching styles is to use your drinks to punctuate little breaks in the conversation, or to give you something to do with your hands. (Unless you're one of those guys who scratches labels off beer bottles; displaying nervous habits with your hands is just as bad as using verbal tics in your speech.) You also want to finish your drink about the same time she finishes hers, so that you can use the ordering of another round as an excuse to hang out together for a while longer. Now you aren't just two strangers who happen to be drinking at the same time in the same place; you're two people having a drink *together*. It's a subtle but important difference.

That, though, brings up another sometimes-tricky issue: who pays. My personal rule is that I don't offer to buy a drink until we've established some quality rapport. I think offering to pay for drinks right off the bat sends the wrong signal. You don't need to trade goods for attention. If she doesn't want to talk to you without a financial commitment on your part, what does that say about the two of you?

Sometimes a woman will ask me to buy her a drink. I try to turn the tables by saying something like, "Buy me one first, and I'll think about it." I like having options, and I hate feeling as if I'm being played—even if the player is the hottest woman in the room. In fact, the more attractive she is, paradoxically, the more important it is to treat her as if she's part of the crowd. Don't be any quicker to buy a drink, and don't try to accelerate the pace of the encounter. Your social value is rising every minute she's in your proximity, so you have no incentive at all to rush things. Plus, the more relaxed you are with her, the more comfortable she's going to feel, which should also work in your favor.

TIP GENEROUSLY

If the encounter has gone on long enough for you to order a couple of drinks together, she's already made some assumptions about your social and financial status. She's looked at your clothes, your haircut, your glasses. She's observed your posture and speech habits. What you drink, as well as how you order it, sends her a message about your preferences, or lack of preferences. Different women are looking for different traits, and if she's still talking to you by the time the check comes, she's decided you're okay, based on what she knows so far. She likes what she sees and what she's heard.

But the way you tip on that first check sends her the first signal about how she might or might not fit into your world. If your clothes or conversational refinement or taste in vodka suggest that you're a guy with some socioeconomic helium, that first tip shows whether or not you're likely to be generous with that money. Lots of the women you meet have worked for tips at some point in their lives. The woman you're chatting up right now might still be working as a waitress or bartender. (Hell, if she's hot, she might work for the kind of tips that get folded up and placed in a G-string.) Chances are, she puts herself in the place of the waiter or bartender presenting you with that first check, and if you don't treat that person right, she's going to take it as a sign that you won't treat her right, either.

Tipping can work for you or against you three different ways:

- If you undertip—giving a buck on a ten-dollar tab, say—it says that you're cheap, or at best insensitive. Either way, you've blown a golden opportunity to show that you're neither of those things.
- If you overtip—putting five dollars on top of that same ten-dollar tab—you could come off as generous, but you could just as easily come off as someone who's trying too hard. A 50 percent tip suggests that you're trying to buy something you can't get any other way. It's sort of like offering to buy her a drink right off the bat, and you'd better believe it has sexual overtones.
- Giving a nitpicky tip—tipping exactly 15 or 20 percent of the tab, and making sure you calculate it right to the nickel—makes you look

like the kind of guy who shelves his books in alphabetical order and counts the number of toilet-paper sheets he uses on each dump. It doesn't matter if that 20 percent tip is relatively generous; you look like either a nerd or a control freak, neither of which suggests that you'll be good in bed.

So what's a good way to tip? First, work with round numbers. If the tab's twelve dollars, throw fifteen dollars onto the bar. You get points for being generous (25 percent) and for not being so nerdy that you ask the bartender for a minuscule amount of change to keep the tip at 20 percent.

But if the tab's thirteen dollars, you're on shakier ground. Throwing fifteen dollars onto the bar gets you points for being casual, but now your tip is just 15 percent, and you're teetering on that chasm separating guys who're generous and cheap. If you have an extra dollar bill, putting it on top of the fifteen dollars shows that you've thought this through, and even though it would be easier to leave it at 15 percent, you don't think that's fair to the bartender. Now you've gone out of your way to be considerate and generous, and all it cost you was a measly dollar.

Group tabs are another chance to show that you're comfortable with money, and by extension with yourself. Don't be the guy who tries to calculate exactly what each person at the table owes based on what they ordered, counting tax and tip. Even worse is developing an uncanny urge to use the john seconds before the check arrives. You might get away with it on a first encounter, but don't expect your friends to stick up for you if you've pulled it more than once.

Let's say you're sitting around a table with five buddies, you're chatting up a group of women, and you're all ready to move on to a new location. The women have already paid for their drinks, and the waitress brings your tab: one hundred dollars, for the six of you. Your best move is to throw twenty dollars on the table, without hesitation. Now you've shown that you're (a) not a nitpicker, since you didn't bother figuring out who owes what, based on what they drank; (b) a decent tipper, since you've calculated a tip into your share of the tab without stopping to think about it; and (c) a man of action, since your twenty-dollar bill hit the table first.

YOU'RE INTERESTED. SHE'S INTERESTED. NOW WHAT?

For all the prep work you did before you went out (including weeks or months of workouts), and for all the consistently encouraging signals you've sent and received, there's really no playbook that teaches you how to proceed when you get to this moment. You know you came here in hopes of meeting someone who'll go home with you. She may have started the evening with the exact same hopes. But now you both have to pretend that this thought of getting naked with each other is occurring to you for the first time.

If you're too eager here, and offer what she perceives as pressure, you'll probably scare her off, even if she started the evening hoping to get to this exact moment with someone much like you.

Each of you will need to tap-dance around this issue of inevitability. How you do that is purely situational. Maybe you say, with reluctance, that you need to accompany your friends to some new locale, making it clear that she and her friends are entirely welcome to join you there. Or maybe the better play is to let her come up with the idea of moving on together. Either way, the dance requires that you somehow convey surprise that your plans for the evening suddenly seem much less important than your desire to spend more time with her. She, in her own way, has to convey a similar dilemma to you. And both of you have to pretend that hooking up wasn't on either of your minds until you met and discovered this mysterious chemistry you seem to share.

The key: you have to be flexible and savvy enough to determine if a first-night hookup is or isn't possible. If she likes you and is interested, however mildly, she's sent you signals to that effect. You hope you've picked up on them. But a lot of extraneous issues go into the decision she's making right now, and most of them probably have nothing to do with you. It doesn't matter if the real problem is physical, psychological, territorial, or familial, or if she feels comfortable telling you her reasons.

If you realize that it's not destined to be a first-night funfest, you have to accept it and decide what happens next. It's your move, and it has to be direct and confident. The smart play is to try to see her again, which means asking for her phone number. But you also have to tell her why you seek the sacred digits. "You want to hang out sometime?" is wimpy. "Let's go out" is unambiguous. It means one thing: "If you give me your phone number, I'll call you and set up a date." Even if she was on the fence about you before, she goes away with a memory of a guy who knows what he wants.

You may or may not be sure you want to follow up, but once you have the phone number, you have the choice. Without it, you don't. (Unless, of course, you have mutual friends or other ways of getting in touch.) She may be just as uncommitted to another encounter with you. When she gives you her number, she forces you to express interest one more time. If you don't call, she may be disappointed, but at least she knows you lost interest as soon as it was clear that she wasn't up for a first-night hookup. If you do call, she still has the option of saying no, and as a bonus (for her) she doesn't have to tell you to your face.

In other words, all the two of you really know when you ask for and receive a phone number is that the possibility of getting together remains open.

Once the digits are scored, however, you're on the clock. But it's a very odd clock, in that it works against you if you call in less than twenty-four hours (you'll seem desperate) or if you wait more than forty-eight hours (you'll seem either callous or calculating). That leaves a twenty-four-hour window in which it's okay to call.

Assuming that you didn't actually make person-to-person contact (and some women, as a habit, won't answer any call if they don't recognize the caller's phone number), that first call puts her on the clock. If she returns it in twenty-four hours or less, she's interested. If she waits more than forty-eight hours, she's not.

Isn't it nice to know that one part of the process is so simple and straightforward?

CHAPTER TWELVE

The End of the Beginning

Halfway through my sophomore year of high school, my friend Kyle took me to the gym and introduced me to my new lifestyle. I was an experienced martial artist and familiar with the concept of "working out," but that day would mark the first time I did something beyond push-ups to build muscle and strength.

We walked to the bench-press station (which, as you know, is the spiritual hub for a generation of lifters) and loaded a twenty-five-pound plate onto each side of the bar. I didn't know a damn thing about training, but I liked the way the heavy weight felt in my hands. I liked the way my body felt after training. Most of all, I liked the idea that, with enough work, I could build a physique good enough to catch the attention of the girls whose looks caught my attention.

So I worked. I lifted. I grunted. I made mistakes. I figured shit out.

After years of trial and error, I finally built that body. The benefits went far beyond what I'd hoped to achieve. Yes, I got the obvious upgrade to my dating life. But I also discovered I had a real passion for learning that had never kicked in when I was in school. (If you don't believe me, ask my former teachers.) The more I learned about strength training and all its related subjects—anatomy, physiology, nutrition, sport-specific conditioning—the more I *wanted* to learn.

From there I discovered I wanted to improve myself in areas that seemed far from the science of building muscles. I wanted to learn about running a business, about writing, about marketing and communication, about being more productive, about leading a healthy and balanced life.

To put it simply, training with weights, and building a lifestyle around my pursuit of a better physique, has taught me more than any professor, mentor, or spiritual guru ever could have.

I think it's because there are no mysteries in the gym. The tools are simple, and they're all out in the open for anyone to use. There are objective criteria. To quote Henry Rollins, "Two hundred pounds will always be two hundred pounds." Either you lift that weight, or you don't. We have to be brutally honest with ourselves. If our perceptions get ahead of our abilities, the iron will put us back in our place.

Just as lessons learned in the gym influenced other parts of my life, I hope you too will discover strengths and personal qualities you never knew you had. For example, you'll almost certainly develop the ability to set meaningful goals and find the resources and ambition you need to achieve them. You'll experience the euphoria of finishing a really challenging workout, even though you wanted to give up before you were halfway through. You'll have evidence that hard work and consistency pay off in the long run, and you'll realize that a quick fix is usually no fix at all. You'll learn the difference between good pain and bad pain. (The first you push through; the second you take as a sign that something has gone wrong, and you act accordingly.) You'll discover how to lose yourself and find yourself, perhaps at the same time.

Most important, no matter what the activity is, you'll learn that you get back as much as you put in. Everything good and lasting is the result of planning, execution, and consistent effort.

As young men, we're constantly branded with stereotypes. We're told we're capable of some things but not others. People want to tell us where we fit in in the world, and where we don't fit. Sometimes these "people" are outsiders, like the media or social scientists. Sometimes they're insiders—family members, friends, coworkers, the girlfriend, the boss. Often, "people" is just one person: you, or me, telling ourselves what we can and can't do.

It takes a lot of practice to master the art of talking back to the narrative, especially if that narrative is inside your own head. There's no simple or straightforward way to do it. Even something that looks easy from the outside—becoming a consistent exerciser and all-around health-conscious guy—can be complicated as hell once you're immersed in the particulars. We all make mistakes, and get frustrated by them. We all backpedal, miss workouts, grab a second slice of cheesecake, fail to make a connection with the hot woman at the bar because our opening comment was embarrassingly lame.

Perfection isn't achievable, and it's not the goal. It's all a learning process. Bruce Lee once said that the only difference between a stumbling block and a stepping-stone is your perception of it. So be careful before you define the challenges you encounter along the way. Figure out where you went wrong. Forgive yourself for making a mistake. And then get back in the game. The only way you lose is if you quit.

Which brings me back to that story about my first-ever bench press. Remember how I told you my friend loaded the bar with a twenty-five on each side? As a lifter, you know that's ninety-five pounds. I lowered it to my chest, but then couldn't raise it an inch. My friend had to pull the bar off my chest. Imagine the humiliation for a high school sophomore, getting pinned by less than one hundred pounds.

I had a choice to make that day. I could either concede that I'd never be a lifter, that a kid who can't even push ninety-five pounds off his chest has no business in the weight room. Or I could make some changes in my approach to exercise. Before long, I was warming up with the weight that had made me feel like the weakest kid in Whitefish, Montana.

That was my choice. What's yours going to be?

RESOURCES AND RECOMMENDED READING

The *Other* Goods

MORE INFORMATION ABOUT *BUILT FOR SHOW*

builtforshow.com

This is a free membership site I've set up exclusively for readers of *Built for Show.* You'll find articles; video demos of every exercise in *BFS,* plus a bunch more. I hope you'll stop by, drop me an e-mail, and let me know how things are going.

ATTRACTION AND SEDUCTION

***Double Your Dating,* by David DeAngelo**

Filled with interesting tidbits on evolutionary psychology and the mating process, David's e-book is the most popular guidebook for aspiring pickup artists.

Rules of the Game, by Neil Strauss

This is Neil's much-anticipated follow-up to *The Game,* the best-seller in which he infiltrated a society of pickup artists and found himself reborn as a first-rate seducer. *Rules of the Game* is a two-book set. The first is a thirty-day challenge for guys, sort of a crash course in the science and practice of hooking up. The second is a collection of some very entertaining short stories.

FASHION

Details: Men's Style Manual, by Daniel Peres

A quick-read fashion guide from the editors at *Details* magazine, with tons of ideas and tips on how to make your clothes work for you and how to create your own style.

FITNESS

T-Nation.com

There's no better place on the Web to find information and advice about training and nutrition from the top experts in the field.

Inside-Out, by Mike Robertson and Bill Hartman

The subtitle calls it "the ultimate upper-body warm-up," but this DVD offers a lot more than that. You'll learn how athletes and lifters can mess up their shoulders, how to figure out the real origins of your own shoulder problems, and how to fix them with a few simple exercises.

Magnificent Mobility, by Eric Cressey and Mike Robertson

The exercises and drills on this exceptional DVD not only improve mobility and flexibility, but also seem to make nagging injuries disappear. At least, that's how it worked for me. You can find it, along with the previous one, at robertsontrainingsystems.com.

Men's Health Power Training, by Robert dos Remedios

Dos is a highly respected strength coach at College of the Canyons in Southern California, where he often has to train dozens of competitive athletes simultaneously. He's always short on time and resources, forcing him to be creative and flexible. Those traits helped him produce a terrific training guide, with twelve-week programs that kicked my ass and lots of exercises I'd never seen before.

The New Rules of Lifting, by Lou Schuler and Alwyn Cosgrove

This is a phenomenal book from two of my most generous and influential mentors. The writing is clear, refreshing, and funny (as only Lou can be), and the workout programs yield amazing results. In fact, *NROL* is a big part of my inspiration for the *Built for Show* workouts. Oh, and if your girlfriend or wife wants to get in shape, have her grab a copy of *The New Rules of Lifting for Women.*

LIFESTYLE

The 4-Hour Workweek, by Timothy Ferriss

Just reading the back flap of *The 4-Hour Workweek*, which reveals that Tim speaks six languages and won a championship in Chinese kickboxing, is enough to motivate you to start living the life of your dreams. I've read the entire book several times.

NUTRITION

Gourmet Nutrition, by John Berardi, Ph.D., Michael Williams, and Kristina Andrew

Let's be honest: a lot of us couldn't find our way around a kitchen with a GPS. John understands, which is why, despite the high-class title, *Gourmet Nutrition* is an outstanding guide to making healthy and tasty meals for yourself and whomever you want to impress on that all-important third date. The directions are simple enough for entry-level kitchen hands to use, and your date never needs to know that the meals are rich in muscle-building protein and low in waist-expanding filler.

Naked Nutrition Guide, by Mike Roussell

Mike, a Ph.D. candidate at Penn State, strips complex nutrition science down to its bare essentials and gives you the information you need to make the right choices and transform your physique while improving your health. I reread this self-published manual every few months to make sure my diet is as dialed-in as it needs to be. You can pick it up at nakednutritionguide.com.

INDEX

alcohol consumption
  drinking styles, 224–25
  guidelines, 201–2
  limits, 20, 37
  paying for drinks, 225
  tipping bartender, 226–27
alternating workouts and
      alternating sets, 49–50
anabolic steroids, 12
attracting women. *See* hooking
      up
availability and approachability,
      219

back-off sets, 77–78
barbell bent-over row, 147
barbell bent-over row with
      underhand grip, 126–27
barbell clean pull, 165
barbell incline bench press,
      148–49
barbell push press, 153–54
barbell reverse curl, 174–75
barbells, sizes and weights of,
      57–59
bench presses
  barbell incline bench press,
      148–49

dumbbell bench press,
      102–4
dumbbell incline bench
      press, 128–29
dumbbell incline bench press
      with neutral grip, 178
  popularity of, 16
biceps curls
  barbell reverse curl, 174–75
  dumbbell alternating curl,
      176–77
  as finisher exercises, 46, 49,
      92
  as isolation exercises, 5–6,
      14–15, 27–28
body-part split epidemic
      (BPSE), 10–12
breads, grains, and cereals,
      189–90
breakfast, 194–95, 196–98
builtforshow.com, 183, 199,
      233
Bulgarian split squat, 137–38
Bulgarian split squat, front foot
      elevated, 169

cable reverse wood chop,
      140–41

cable row, wide-grip, 99–101
cable row with neutral grip,
      155–56
cable wood chop, 122–23
calories, 25, 29, 194
carbohydrates, 28, 29, 196
cardio workouts, 49, 92
cereals, grains, and breads,
      189–90
charts. *See* workout charts
chin-up, 105–6
condiments, 190–91
confidence, 211–13
conversation, 222–23
Cosgrove, Alwyn, 212
crunches
  reverse crunch, 111
  Swiss-ball crunch, 151
curls
  barbell reverse curl, 174–75
  dumbbell alternating curl,
      176–77
  as finisher exercises, 46, 49, 92
  as isolation exercises, 5–6,
      14–15, 27–28

dairy foods and eggs, 187–88
dating. *See* hooking up

deadlifts
  barbell clean pull, 165
  deadlift, 135–36
  dumbbell Romanian deadlift, 144
DeAngelo, David, 42
diet. *See* foods and diet
dip (exercise), 132–34
dos Remedios, Robert, 70
dressing guidelines
  general rules, 204–6
  for heavy guys, 209–10
  recommended reading, 234
  for skinny guys, 207–9
drinks
  drinking styles, 224–25
  guidelines, 201–2
  limits, 20, 37
  paying for, 225
  tipping bartender, 226–27
dumbbell alternating curl, 176–77
dumbbell bench press, 102–4
dumbbell hang snatch, 157–58
dumbbell incline bench press, 128–29
dumbbell incline bench press with neutral grip, 178
dumbbell lying triceps extension, 179
dumbbell Romanian deadlift, 144
dumbbell shoulder press, 150
dumbbell shoulder press with neutral grip, 109–10
dumbbells, types and brands of, 103

eating. *See* foods and diet; meal plan
eggs and dairy foods, 187–88
exercise machines, 5
expectations and mind-sets
  controllable factors, 24
  of fat guys, 28–30
  genetic limitations, 20–22, 30
  of skinny guys, 25–28
eye contact, 223

failure, lifting to, 60–61
Fall workout
  goals and features, 8, 48, 72–73
  Phase 1 charts, 73–75
  Phase 2 charts, 75–77
fashion
  general rules, 204–6
  for heavy guys, 209–10
  recommended reading, 234
  for skinny guys, 207–9
fat guys
  fashion rules, 204–6, 209–10
  mind-set, 28–30
fat loss
  interval training for, 49
  regular meals, 28
  Spring and Summer workouts, 48, 87, 92
  total-body training versus isolation exercises, 14
finisher exercises, 46, 49, 92
fish, 187
fitness resources, 234–35
flexibility versus mobility, 68
foods and diet. *See also* meal plan
  breakfast suggestions, 196–98
  calories, 25, 29, 194
  carbohydrate/protein combination, 28, 29, 196
  condiments, 190–91
  dairy and eggs, 187–88
  fast food, 33
  fish, 187
  fruits and vegetables, 188–89
  grains, cereals, breads, 189–90
  healthy diet, 19–20, 32–33, 184–85
  label reading, 192–93
  nutrition resources, 235–36
  poor nutrition, 30–31
  poultry, 186–87
  recipe resource, 183, 199

red meat, 185–86
  supplements, 19, 198
front squat, 114–16
front squat to push press, 166–67
fruits and vegetables, 188–89

genetic factors, 20–22, 30
glutes, attractiveness of, 44–45
goblet squat, 139
grains, cereals, and breads, 189–90
gym equipment, 57–59, 103

habits. *See* lifestyle
hard gainers, 25
Hartman, Bill, 67
heavy guys
  fashion rules, 204–6, 209–10
  mind-set, 28–30
hooking up
  attractive physique, 16–17, 42–46
  availability and approachability, 219
  confidence, 211–13
  conversation, 222–23
  eye contact, 223
  first move, 220–21
  first-night hookup, 228
  incidental contact, 224
  leaning forward, 224
  matching drinking styles, 224–25
  paying for drinks, 225
  phone number exchange, 229
  posture, 217–18
  preparation for, 218–19
  recognizing signs of interest, 220
  resources on, 233–34
  standards, 216–17
  tipping at bar, 226
hormones
  boost from total-body workouts, 15, 49
  hormonal warm-up, 55
  release during sleep, 32

intervals, 49, 92, 95
isolation exercises
　in addition to total-body
　　exercises, 15
　body-part split epidemic
　　(BPSE), 10–12
　as finisher exercises, 46, 49,
　　92
　futility of, 5–6, 11–14,
　　27–28

John, Dan, 31
joint mobility
　vs. flexibility, 68
　importance of, 66–67
　lateral over-under drill, 70
　leg swings, 69
　T push-up, 71
jump lunge, 168
jump squat, 160–61

KFC syndrome, 17

lat pulldown, underhand-grip,
　107–8
lat pulldown, wide-grip,
　130–31
lat pulldown with neutral grip,
　172–73
lateral over-under drill, 70
Lee, Bruce, 232
leg swings, 69
lifestyle
　diet, 32–33
　recommended reading on,
　　235
　sleep, 31–32
　time-wasting, 34–37
　unhealthy habits, 30–31
　workout routine, 33–34
lifting. See seasonal workout
　program
log, training, 62–65
lower-body routines
　Fall Phase 1 workout B,
　　74–75
　Fall Phase 2 workout B,
　　76–77

Winter Phase 1 workout
　A, 80
Winter Phase 1 workout
　C, 81
Winter Phase 2 workout
　A, 83
Winter Phase 2 workout
　C, 85
lunges
　jump lunge, 168
　reverse lunge, 145–46

machine exercises, 5
meal plan. See also foods and
　diet
　breakfast, 194–95, 196
　eating schedule, 28, 33,
　　193–96, 200–201
　guidelines, 191–93
　lunch and dinner, 199–200
　postworkout nutrition, 28,
　　195–96, 198–99
　preworkout meals, 28
　snacks, 200
meat and poultry, 185–87
metabolism boost
　from calories consumed, 25,
　　29, 194
　front squat to push press,
　　166–67
　jump squat, 160–61
　from muscle-building
　　process, 30
　from total-body workouts,
　　15, 48
midsection, attractiveness of, 45
mobility
　vs. flexibility, 68
　importance of, 66–67
　lateral over-under drill, 70
　leg swings, 69
　T push-up, 71
muscle development
　attractive physique, 16–17,
　　42–46
　calories for, 25, 194
　flexibility, 68
　hard gainers, 25

isolation exercises, 10–15,
　27–28, 46, 49
metabolism boost, 30
vs. pump, 5–6, 26
during rest, 32, 53
strength, 17, 26–27
through total-body training,
　13–15
tone and definition, 25–26
vanity, 16–17
Mystery (pickup artist), 220

nutrition. See foods and diet;
　meal plan
nutritional supplements, 19,
　198

Olympic barbells and weight
　plates, 57–59

periodized workout program,
　47, 51–52
PHAT warm-ups, 55–57
phone number, asking for, 229
physique, attractive, 16–17,
　42–46
picking up women. See hooking
　up
planks
　plank, 112–13
　side plank, 124–25
　3-point plank, 159
posture, 18, 217–18
postworkout nutrition, 28,
　195–96, 198–99
poultry, 186–87
presses
　barbell incline bench press,
　　148–49
　barbell push press, 153–54
　dumbbell bench press,
　　102–4
　dumbbell incline bench
　　press, 128–29
　dumbbell incline bench press
　　with neutral grip, 178
　dumbbell shoulder press,
　　150

presses (*cont.*)
  dumbbell shoulder press with neutral grip, 109–10
  front squat to push press, 166–67
  single-arm push press, 163–64
preworkout meals, 28
program. *See* seasonal workout program
protein
  with carbohydrates, 28, 29, 196
  dairy and eggs, 187–88
  fish, 187
  in fruits and vegetables, 188
  postworkout nutrition, 195–96, 198–99
  poultry, 186–87
  preworkout meals, 28
  red meat, 185–86
psychological warm-up, 55
pulldowns
  lat pulldown with neutral grip, 172–73
  underhand-grip lat pulldown, 107–8
  wide-grip lat pulldown, 130–31
pull-up, wide-grip, 162
pump of muscles, 5–6, 25–26, 218
push-ups
  push-up, 170
  rock-climber push-up, 171
  T push-up, 71

red meat, 185–86
rest and recovery, 32, 53–54
reverse crunch, 111
reverse lunge, 145–46
rock-climber push-up, 171
Rollins, Henry, 231
routines. *See* lifestyle; workout charts
rowing exercises
  barbell bent-over row, 147

barbell bent-over row with underhand grip, 126–27
cable row with neutral grip, 155–56
wide-grip cable row, 99–101

seasonal workout program. *See also specific seasons*
  alternating workouts and alternating sets, 49–50
  amount of weight to use, 59–60
  goals, 8
  lifting to failure, 60–61
  number of workouts per week, 48
  periodization, 47, 51–52
  rest and recovery, 53–54
  speed of lifting, 62
  split routines, 48
  total-body training, 48–49
  training log, 62–65
  undulating periodization, 51–52
  warm-up, 55–57
  workout charts, to use, 49–52
self-confidence, 211–13
shakes, postworkout, 195–96, 198
shoulder press, dumbbell, 150
shoulder press, dumbbell with neutral grip, 109–10
shoulders, attractiveness of, 44
side plank, 124–25
single-arm push press, 163–64
skinny guys
  fashion rules, 204–9
  mind-set, 25–28
skinny-fat guys
  diet, 30–31, 32–33
  sleep, 31–32
  use of time, 34–37
  workout routine, 33–34
sleep, 31–32
Smith machine, 58–59

snacks, 200
snatch, dumbbell hang, 157–58
speed of lifting, 62
split routines, 48. *See also* lower-body routines; upper-body routines
Spring workout
  goals and features, 8, 48–49, 86–87
  Phase 1 charts, 88–89
  Phase 2 charts, 90–91
sprints, 92, 94
squats
  Bulgarian split squat, 137–38
  Bulgarian split squat, front foot elevated, 169
  front squat, 114–16
  front squat to push press, 166–67
  goblet squat, 139
  jump squat, 160–61
  squat, 142–43
standards for dating, 216–17
step-up, 117–18
steroids, 12
Strauss, Neil, 215
strength, 17, 26–27
style. *See* fashion
Summer workout
  goals and features, 8, 48–49, 92
  Phase 1 charts, 93–95
  Phase 2 charts, 96–98
supine hip extension/leg curl, 119–21
supplements, 19, 198
Swiss-ball crunch, 151

T push-up, 71
technical warm-up, 56–57
3-point plank, 159
time-wasting habit, 34–37
tipping of bartender, 226–27
total-body routines
  Spring Phase 1 workout A, 88

Spring Phase 1 workout B, 89

Spring Phase 2 workout A, 90

Spring Phase 2 workout B, 91

Summer Phase 1 workout A, 93–94

Summer Phase 1 workout B, 94–95

Summer Phase 2 workout A, 96–97

Summer Phase 2 workout B, 97–98

total-body training. *See also* Spring workout; Summer workout

balanced workouts, 17–18

benefits, 13–15

goals and features, 48–49

training log, 62–65

training program. *See* seasonal workout program

triceps extension

dumbbell lying triceps extension, 179

as finisher exercise, 49, 92

underhand-grip lat pulldown, 107–8

undulating periodization, 51–52

upper-body routines

Fall Phase 1 workout A, 73–74

Fall Phase 2 workout A, 75–76

Winter Phase 1 workout B, 80–81

Winter Phase 1 workout D, 82

Winter Phase 2 workout B, 84

Winter Phase 2 workout D, 86

vegetables and fruits, 188–89

warm-ups

lateral over-under drill, 70

leg swings, 69

for mobility, 66–68

T push-up, 71

variables, 55–57

wave loading, 78–79

Web site, builtforshow.com, 183, 199, 233

weight loss. *See* fat loss

weights

amount to lift, 59–60

gym equipment, 57–59, 103

wide-grip cable row, 99–101

wide-grip lat pulldown, 130–31

wide-grip pull-up, 162

Winter workout

goals and features, 8, 48, 77–79

Phase 1 charts, 80–82

Phase 2 charts, 83–86

women, attracting. *See* hooking up

workout charts

Fall Phase 1 workout A, 73–74

Fall Phase 1 workout B, 74–75

Fall Phase 2 workout A, 75–76

Fall Phase 2 workout B, 76–77

Spring Phase 1 workout A, 88

Spring Phase 1 workout B, 89

Spring Phase 2 workout A, 90

Spring Phase 2 workout B, 91

Summer Phase 1 workout A, 93–94

Summer Phase 1 workout B, 94–95

Summer Phase 2 workout A, 96–97

Summer Phase 2 workout B, 97–98

Winter Phase 1 workout A, 80

Winter Phase 1 workout B, 80–81

Winter Phase 1 workout C, 81

Winter Phase 1 workout D, 82

Winter Phase 2 workout A, 83

Winter Phase 2 workout B, 84

Winter Phase 2 workout C, 85

Winter Phase 2 workout D, 86

workout goals and pitfalls, 3–6

workout program. *See* seasonal workout program